CANCER PREVENTION
RESEARCH TRENDS

CANCER PREVENTION RESEARCH TRENDS

LOUIS BRAUN
AND
MAXIMILIAN LANGE
EDITORS

Nova Science Publishers, Inc.
New York

For permission to use material from this book please contact us:
Telephone 631-231-7269; Fax 631-231-8175
Web Site: http://www.novapublishers.com

NOTICE TO THE READER

The Publisher has taken reasonable care in the preparation of this book, but makes no expressed or implied warranty of any kind and assumes no responsibility for any errors or omissions. No liability is assumed for incidental or consequential damages in connection with or arising out of information contained in this book. The Publisher shall not be liable for any special, consequential, or exemplary damages resulting, in whole or in part, from the readers' use of, or reliance upon, this material.

Independent verification should be sought for any data, advice or recommendations contained in this book. In addition, no responsibility is assumed by the publisher for any injury and/or damage to persons or property arising from any methods, products, instructions, ideas or otherwise contained in this publication.

This publication is designed to provide accurate and authoritative information with regard to the subject matter covered herein. It is sold with the clear understanding that the Publisher is not engaged in rendering legal or any other professional services. If legal or any other expert assistance is required, the services of a competent person should be sought. FROM A DECLARATION OF PARTICIPANTS JOINTLY ADOPTED BY A COMMITTEE OF THE AMERICAN BAR ASSOCIATION AND A COMMITTEE OF PUBLISHERS.

Library of Congress Cataloging-in-Publication Data

Cancer prevention research trends / Louis Braun and Maximilian Lange, editors.
  p. ; cm.
 Includes bibliographical references and index.
 ISBN 978-1-60456-639-0 (hardcover)
 1. Cancer--Prevention. I. Braun, Louis, 1951- II. Lange, Maximilian.
 [DNLM: 1. Biomedical Research--trends. 2. Neoplasms--prevention & control. QZ 206 C2149 2008]
  RC268.C3657 2008
  362.196'994--dc22
                         2008013822

Published by Nova Science Publishers, Inc. ✦ New York

Contents

Preface   **ix**

Chapter I   Direct-to-Consumer-Advertising Exposure
Impedes Lifestyle-Focused Cancer Prevention Efforts   **1**
Dominick L. Frosch

Chapter II   Gastric, Colorectal and Pancreatic Carcinoma: The Relationship
between Hemostasis and Cancer Prognostic Markers   **5**
Hussain Alizadeh, Shaikhah Al-Tajer, and Shaker A. Mousa

Chapter III   Vitamin D Use among Older Adults in U.S.:
Results from National Surveys 1997 To 2002   **21**
Euni Lee, Mary Maneno, Anthony K. Wutoh and Seok-Woo Lee

Chapter IV   Paricalcitol: A Vitamin D2 Analog
with Anticancer Effects with Low Calcemic Activity   **39**
Takashi Kumagai and H. Phillip Koeffler

Chapter V   Reduction in the Risk of Human Breast Cancer by Selective
Cyclooxygenase-2 (COX-2) Inhibitors:
Final Results of a Case Control Study   **51**
Randall E. Harris, Joanne Beebe-Donk and Galal A. Alshafie

Chapter VI   Counseling Undergraduates of the Health Care Professions in a
Developing Country: Are there Peculiar Needs or Desires?   **61**
*Olayinka. O. Omigbodun, Akinyinka. O. Omigbodun,
and Akin-Tunde A. Odukogbe*

Chapter VII   Alternative Approaches to Cervical Cancer Prevention:
Risk-Adapted Multimodal Laboratory Cervical Screening   **99**
*Reinhard Bollmann, Alinda Dalma Varnai, Agnes Bankfalvi
and Magdolna Bollmann*

Chapter VIII   Can a Home-Visit Invitation Increase Pap Smear Screening
in Samliem, Khon Kaen, Thailand?   **113**
W. Chalapati and B. Chumworathayi

Index   **125**

Preface

Cancer has a complex etiology, probably due to a sophisticated interaction between the genetic endowment of individuals and environmental risk factors. The continuing magnitude and severity of cancer as a major health problem renders cancer prevention an important area in the field of cancer research. Developments in cancer prevention have benefitted from the recent advances in molecular and cellular biology. Several specific molecules have been identified as promising targets for cancer prevention and numerous agents have been synthesized, developed and tested to modulate the functions of these molecules. Given the ongoing advances in our understanding in the genesis of cancer, it is possible to develop new and better agents on a more mechanistic basis. The most striking examples for this mechanism-based approach for cancer prevention include: the role of inducible cyclooxygenase-2 (COX-2) in colon cancer and the preventive effects of COX-2 inhibitors (e.g., celecoxib); the involvement of estrogen receptors in breast cancer and the development of selective estrogen receptor modulators (e.g., tamoxifen and raloxifene) for the prevention of this malignancy; and the function of androgen in prostate cancer and the use of 5-á-reductase inhibitors (e.g., finasteride) as a preventive measure. This new book brings together important research from around the world in this challenging field.

Chapter I - Communication is a central component of primary cancer prevention efforts. In 1997 the FDA clarified its regulations governing direct-to-consumer-advertising (DTCA) of prescription pharmaceutical products making television advertising feasible for the first time. Spending on this type of marketing has grown tremendously and many Americans are exposed to a high number of pharmaceutical ads. Little is known about the broader effects of this exposure. DTCA for pharmaceuticals appears to promote the meta-message that these products will solve all health problems, including cancer. Repeated exposure to these ads may render attempts to encourage lifestyle modification to prevent cancer less effective.

Chapter II - Patients with different types of nonhematological, solid organ tumor (esophageal adenocarcinoma, gastric cancer, colorectal cancer, exocrine pancreatic adenocarcinoma, or adenocarcinoma of gallbladder) were studied. Detailed monitoring upon admission and prior to any cancer-related intervention and on a weekly basis post-intervention (chemotherapy, radiation or surgery) but not anticoagulant for up to 18 weeks were carried out. Natural inhibitors of coagulation (protein C, protein S, and antithrombin), and D-dimer and prothrombin activation peptide F1+2 as markers of the status of fibrinolytic and coagulation systems were determined. In all cases the levels of hypercoagulable markers were elevated directly correlated with tumor markers and radiological findings. Additionally, the level of naturally occurring coagulation inhibitors all decreased with tumor progression. Thus, determination of hemostasis activation state can be used to assess the tumor prognosis, and early anticoagulation prophylaxis might prevent venous thromboembolism and impair tumor progression.

Chapter III – Osteoporosis is the most common bone disease leading to increased fracture risk and is associated with permanent disability and poor outcomes. Established guidelines emphasize the role of calcium/vitamin D supplementation for optimal management of osteoporosis. Current literature indicates under-diagnosis with osteoporosis, and under-use of anti-osteoporosis medications with calcium/vitamin D supplementation upon diagnosis. Few studies have evaluated utilization patterns and trends of vitamin D among the older US population for prevention and/or treatment, and even fewer studies have assessed the prevalence of vitamin D use evaluating national level databases. Therefore, this study was conducted to evaluate recent trends in vitamin D prescribing using two national databases; the National Ambulatory Medical Care Survey (NAMCS) and Medical Expenditure Panel Survey (MEPS) from 1997 to 2002. NAMCS is an annual survey conducted by the National Center for Health Statistics (NCHS). The Agency for Healthcare Research and Quality (AHRQ) conducts MEPS in conjunction with the NCHS. NAMCS and MEPS are important resources designed to provide information about health care use and costs (MEPS only) in the U.S. as indicated by visits made by non-institutionalized patients and individuals drawn from a nationally representative sub-sample of households across the nation. This study provides 6-year trends in vitamin D use, characteristics of individuals that are associated with vitamin D, and predictors of vitamin D prescribing. Our findings indicated that very few visits made by patients were associated with vitamin D prescriptions. The overall utilization of vitamin D therapy in the U.S. between1997 and 2002 was suboptimal. Older and female patients, and patients with an osteoporosis diagnosis were more likely to be receiving vitamin D therapy. Our findings support the need for greater awareness regarding vitamin D supplementation among patients who are 40 years and older, especially among male patients, through patient counseling. A coordinated effort and comprehensive programmatic approach among health care professional including physicians, dentists, nurses, pharmacists, and nutritionists are recommended to improve osteoporosis prevention and treatment.

Chapter IV - The use of *all-trans*-retinoic acid (ATRA) for the treatment of acute promyelocytic leukemia shows the power of a non-chemotherapeutic drug to induce the terminal differentiation of leukemia cells. Vitamin D compounds also inhibit the growth of various types of cancers by inducing their differentiation and inhibiting their proliferation *in vitro and vivo*. In a clinical study, orally administered $1,25(OH)_2D_3$ had modest usefullness for pre-leukemic patients. Because of the calcemic side-effect of $1,25(OH)_2D_3$, the dosage that could be given to these individuals was less than theoretically required for an anticancer effect as noted in vitro. Therefore, new potent, but less calcemic analogs of vitamin D are being synthesized and tested. $19\text{-}nor\text{-}1,25(OH)_2D_2$ (Paricalcitol) is a synthetic analogue of $1,25(OH)_2D_2$ currently approved by the FDA for the clinical treatment of secondary hyperparathyroidism in patients with chronic renal failure. This compound has very little calcemic potential as shown by several controlled, randomized clinical trials. Notably, the antiproliferative effects of $19\text{-}nor\text{-}1,25(OH)_2D_2$ against human cancers have also recently been reported, including activity against prostate and colon cancers, as well as leukemia and multiple myeloma cells *in vitro* and *in vivo,* associated with cell cycle arrest, induction of differentiation and apoptosis, as well as, decreased expression levels of some tumor suppressor genes. The effect of the analog is mediated through the vitamin D receptor. A clinical trial of paricalcitol has been performed in patients with myelodysplastic syndrome (MDS). Although this therapy was not toxic and hypercalcemia was rarely detected, overall it was not very effective, suggesting that the vitamin vitamin D analog alone may need to be combined with other clinicaly useful drugs.

The combination of vitamin D compounds with other agents have been examined including the addition of the inhibitor of the mitochondrial enzyme, $1,25(OH)_2D_3$ 24-hydroxylase. It is a transcriptional target gene of vitamin D and catalyzes the initial step in the conversion of the active molecule $1,25(OH)_2D_3$ into the less potent metabolite, $1,24,25(OH)_2D_3$. Another example is arsenic trioxide. We have reported that paricalcitol in combination with arsenic trioxide has markedly enhanced anti-myeloid leukemia activity in vitro compared to either agent alone. This may be the case because arsenic trioxide acts as an inhibitor of both 24-hydroxylase as well as the PML-RARα fusion protein, the leukemogenic fusion protein that represses normal blood cell differentiation in this leukemia.

In summary, vitamin D analogs alone may not be potent enough to become a viable anticancer therapy; but when combined with other compounds, they may provide a therapeutic approach to cancers with little toxicity.

Chapter V - Background: Epidemiologic and laboratory investigations suggest that nonsteroidal anti-inflammatory drugs (NSAIDs) have chemopreventive effects against breast cancer due to their activity against cyclooxygenase-2 (COX-2), the rate-limiting enzyme of the prostaglandin cascade.

Methods: The authors conducted a case control study of breast cancer designed to compare effects of selective and non-selective COX-2 inhibitors. A total of 611 incident breast cancer patients were ascertained from the James Cancer Hospital, Columbus, Ohio, during 2003-2004 and compared with 615 cancer free controls frequency-matched to the cases on age, race, and county of residence. Data on the past and current use of prescription and over the counter medications and breast cancer risk factors were ascertained using a standardized risk factor questionnaire. Effects of COX-2 inhibiting agents were quantified by calculating odds ratios (OR) and 95% confidence intervals.

Results: Results showed significant risk reductions for selective COX-2 inhibitors as a group (OR=0.15, 95% CI=0.08-0.28), regular aspirin (OR=0.46, 95% CI = 0.32-0.65), and ibuprofen or naproxen (0.36, 95% CI= 0.21-0.60). Intake of COX-2 inhibitors produced significant risk reductions for premenopausal women (OR=0.05), postmenopausal women (OR=0.26), women with a positive family history (OR=0.19), women with a negative family history (OR=0.14), women with estrogen receptor positive tumors (OR=0.24), women with estrogen receptor negative tumors (OR=0.05), women with HER-2/neu positive tumors (OR=0.26), and women with HER-2/neu negative tumors (OR=0.17). Acetaminophen, a compound with negligible COX-2 activity produced no significant change in the risk of breast cancer.

Conclusions: Selective COX-2 inhibitors (celecoxib and rofecoxib) were only recently approved for use in 1999, and rofecoxib (Vioxx) was withdrawn from the marketplace in 2004. Nevertheless, even in the short window of exposure to these compounds, the selective COX-2 inhibitors produced a significant (85%) reduction in the risk of breast cancer, underscoring their strong potential for breast cancer chemoprevention.

Chapter VI - For many students, university life is extremely stressful. However studies suggest that undergraduates in the health care professions have peculiar stresses due to long hours of study and longer duration of study. Nigeria is a typical example of a developing country with all the problems of basic infrastructure. This implies that health care students may have to deal with stress not only from their course of study, but also from having to cope with living in a developing world context. Structured counseling services may help but are yet to be put in place. In developing counseling services, it is important to carry out a needs-assessment to identify what the students perceive their requirements to be.

This study utilizes both quantitative and qualitative methods to look into the circumstances the students recognize would require counseling, and also the type of facility desired. Having obtained informed consent from them, 1118 students of medicine, dentistry, physiotherapy and nursing, completed questionnaires about their counseling needs and what they consider desirable in a counseling facility.

Twelve themes emerged as circumstances requiring counseling: academic problems, courtship and marriage issues, future career, financial problems, emotional problems, family problems, spiritual problems and issues of religion, problems with physical health, difficult teachers, problems with utilities (accommodation, transport, catering and related issues), sexual harassment, and alcohol/drug use.

Some of the conditions desired by the students for a counseling service were confidentiality, counselors with a 'good attitude', enlightenment campaigns, made optional for students, affordability and accessibility, and provision of a 24-hour service. Other features desired were a combined counseling service offered by professionals and lecturers, wide service coverage to include areas such as academic, emotional and spiritual counseling. There should also be sensitivity to ethnicity, culture and religious affiliation.

Undergraduates in their first year were more likely to request counseling for academic and emotional or psychological problems while students in their final year were more likely to request counseling about future careers and difficulty with teachers. Females were more likely to request counseling for academic problems while the males seemed to be more concerned with emotional and financial problems. The females required counseling as an avenue to ventilate and were particularly concerned about confidentiality while the males required it for decision making. Students showing evidence of psychological distress had a significantly different pattern of need for counseling in the areas of academic difficulties, emotional problems, finances and problems with utilities

The findings demonstrate that the counseling needs in these undergraduates are similar to what obtains in other parts of the world, although there are some needs, notably in the area of spiritual and religious issues, that derive from the developing country environment in which they are studying.

Chapter VII - Cervical screening is acknowledged as currently the most effective approach for cervical cancer control. To date, there is extensive and strong evidence that cytology-based screening programs have been effective in reducing the incidence of and mortality from the disease in developed countries. However, conventional Papanicolaou (Pap) smears have inherent methodological shortcomings. New developments in cytology, such as liquid-based techniques and automated reading, seem to effectively overcome some of these limitations and have the potential to improve sensitivity and specificity of cytology both in diagnosis of and screening for cervical pre-cancer and cancer.

The recognition that cervical cancer is a consequence of an acquired infection with a few types of oncogenic human papillomaviruses (HPV) has led to novel opportunities for screening based on the use of HPV-tests. Current HPV testing systems are able to detect the presence of viral DNA in exfoliated cervical epithelial cells in close to 100% of invasive cervical cancer and up to 90% of its precursors. Thus, in terms of public health and also for practical purposes, all cervical cancer cases should be considered to be caused by HPV infection. A number of clinical studies have also demonstrated HPV testing to be more sensitive for the detection of clinically relevant pre-invasive cervical disease than cytology alone and the combination of HPV tests and cytology may achieve a negative predictive value of >97% in detecting high grade intraepithelial neoplasia and cervical cancer.

However, in most women, cervical HPV infections remain asymptomatic and are transient, becoming undetectable in 1-2 years even by the most sensitive genetic tests. This is also true for high-risk HPV (HR-HPV) types. It is the long term persistence of certain HR-HPV genotypes that is strongly associated with cervical carcinogenesis in permissive cases. Therefore, discrimination between transient and persistent infections with a certain HPV genotype is essential for risk-adapted screening protocols, which can only be defined by genotyping of two consecutive probes.

Nevertheless, even the highly sensitive test combination of cytology and HR-HPV genotyping cannot predict the biological potential of prevalent cervical pre-cancers towards progression or regression. This can only be assessed by using an adequate biomarker of neoplastic transformation, e.g., DNA aneuploidy, in combination with morphological and HPV tests.

This review focuses on the clinical utility of conventional, ancillary and experimental methods for cervical screening and possible future directions for enhanced screening accuracy and prognostication using risk-adapted multimodal protocols.

Chapter VIII - Objective: To assess the efficiency of a home-visit invitation aimed to increase uptake of cervical cancer screening in women between 35 and 60 years of age.

Method: Since May, 2006, the authors conducted a quasi-randomized trial to determine if an in-home education and invitation intervention would increase uptake of cervical cancer screening. The authors randomly recruited 304 women from the Samliem inner-city community, Khon Kaen, Northeast Thailand, and assigned participants to either the intervention or control zone. Baseline screening coverage interviews were then done: 58 of 158 women in the intervention zone and 46 of 146 in the control zone were excluded from the study because of having had a Pap smear within 5 years, but these were included in the final analysis. First, 100 women in the intervention group were visited in their homes by one of the researchers, who provided culturally-sensitive health education that emphasized the need for screening. Four months later, post-intervention, screening-coverage interviews were again performed in both groups, in combination with the same health education for 100 women in the control group for a comparison.

Results: There was no difference in the baseline Pap smear screening-coverage rate in the intervention *vs.* control zones (36.7 *vs.* 31.5%, p=0.339). One hundred women in the intervention group completed the intervention interviews and after four months, 100 women in the intervention group and 100 in the control group also completed the post-intervention interviews. The increased screening-coverage rate in the intervention zone was similar to that of the control zone (43.6 *vs.* 34.9%, p=0.119); however, there was a borderline significant increase in the intervention zone compared with baseline (36.7 to 43.6%, p=0.070).

Conclusion: Home visit education and invitation intervention produced a borderline significant effect on increasing Pap smear coverage within 4 months of study period.

In: Cancer Prevention Research Trends
Editors: Louis Braun and Maximilian Lange

ISBN: 978-1-60456-639-0
© 2008 Nova Science Publishers, Inc.

Chapter I

Direct-to-Consumer-Advertising Exposure Impedes Lifestyle-Focused Cancer Prevention Efforts

Dominick L. Frosch[*]
University of Pennsylvania

Abstract

Communication is a central component of primary cancer prevention efforts. In 1997 the FDA clarified its regulations governing direct-to-consumer-advertising (DTCA) of prescription pharmaceutical products making television advertising feasible for the first time. Spending on this type of marketing has grown tremendously and many Americans are exposed to a high number of pharmaceutical ads. Little is known about the broader effects of this exposure. DTCA for pharmaceuticals appears to promote the meta-message that these products will solve all health problems, including cancer. Repeated exposure to these ads may render attempts to encourage lifestyle modification to prevent cancer less effective.

KeyWords: direct-to-consumer-advertising, pharmaceuticals, cancer prevention.

Coinciding with the 2004 Tour de France cycling race, in which Lance Armstrong achieved the unprecedented feat of sixth consecutive victory, Bristol-Myers Squibb broadcast an advertisement on television that has played before. In the ad Mr. Armstrong briefly sketches the story of his own battle with testicular cancer, deservedly crediting his remission to cancer drugs developed by Bristol-Myers Squibb. In the final moments of the ad that shows researchers working in a laboratory, viewers hear the promise of "hope, triumph, and the miracle of medicine". Although this ad was not for a particular product, it is part of a

[*] Correspondence: Dominick Frosch, Robert Wood Johnson Health and Society Scholar, Senior Fellow, Leonard Davis Institute of Health Economics, University of Pennsylvania, 3641 Locust Walk, Philadelphia, PA 19104, frosch@wharton.upenn.edu

larger marketing campaign for prescription pharmaceuticals that may have important effects on cancer prevention efforts in the US. "Triumph" and "miracle" are powerful words that can evoke strong feelings of hope in fighting cancer. By contrast, behaviors that are promoted to prevent cancer are neither triumphant nor miraculous and rarely if ever offer simple solutions. They often demand tedious effort from those that attempt to engage in these important behavioral changes. Yet, effective population-based cancer control requires continued reductions in tobacco smoking, animal fat intake, increased physical activity and intake of fruits and vegetables, as well as limited alcohol use and safe sexual practices [1].

Pharmaceutical ads have been running on the airwaves of American television since 1997 when the FDA clarified its "adequate provision rule" [2]. This rule requires that any ad marketing a prescription product include a summary of information regarding product side effects, warnings, precautions, and contraindications. Prior to 1997 providing this information in a broadcast ad posed a substantial and potentially costly challenge, effectively keeping ads off the airwaves [3]. The FDA clarification stated that broadcast advertisements could meet the requirements of the adequate provision rule by referring consumers to a toll-free telephone number, a healthcare provider, a concurrent print ad, or an Internet web page to obtain more detailed product information. This significantly reduced the amount of broadcast time required to comply with FDA regulations [2]. As a result, spending by pharmaceutical companies on direct-to-consumer-advertising (DTCA) has grown dramatically and is expected to reach a staggering $7.5 billion by 2005 [4, 5].

The effects of this increase in advertising are profound. Few Americans have not seen such ads and one estimate suggests that the average television viewer is exposed to as many as nine ads per day [6]. Pharmaceutical sales figures from recent years suggest that DTCA achieves industry's desired effect [4]. DTCA spending tends to be concentrated in a small number of products. In 1999 24 brands accounted for 74% of DTCA spending. These 24 brands had a 42% increase in sales in 1999, compared to 14.4% for all other drugs on the market. Overall, these 24 brands accounted for 34% of the increase in pharmaceutical spending between 1998 and 1999 [7]. It has been estimated that every dollar spent on television DTCA returns $1.69 in pharmaceutical sales [6]. A recent study examined the impact of DTCA on patient requests for drugs and physician prescribing practices in Sacramento, California, and Vancouver, Canada [8]. Although Canada does not permit DTCA of pharmaceutical products, individuals living in Vancouver were nevertheless exposed to DTCA through watching US-based broadcasts, albeit at significantly lower levels than those living in Sacramento. Findings indicated that patients in Sacramento were twice as likely as patients in Vancouver to request a prescription for an advertised drug.

Beyond patient requests for specific prescriptions, there are important questions about broader cumulative effects of DTCA exposure [9]. For such effects to occur the first question is whether all the exposure generated by DTCA promotes a consistent message. On the surface this might not appear to be the case. The ads we see on television are for a range of products for conditions that range from relatively benign to potentially life-threatening. The specific marketing messages necessarily vary to some degree from product to product. Nevertheless, there appears to be a meta-message in DTCA that goes beyond the manifest content of the ads. All drug marketing campaigns share the goal of increasing sales of the advertised product [10]. In pursuing this goal they aim to convince consumers that their products are superior, often by characterizing them as novel. Given its emphasis on increasing pharmaceutical product sales, DTCA emphasizes the use of medication in addressing health problems. Anecdotal impressions suggest that in promoting products, DTCA tends to emphasize cures and breakthroughs. Given evidence indicating that people substantially overestimate the effectiveness of advertised products, the meta-message of DTCA may lead people to believe that pharmaceutical products or healthcare services will solve all health problems [11]. This meta-message may have important effects that extend beyond the indication for a given product, especially among those with limited exposure to the healthcare system and its inherent uncertainties. It may lead people to spend less time thinking about and engaging in healthy lifestyle choices and preventative behavior in considering their own cancer risk. It could further suggest that even if a behavior contributes to cancer, products will be available to counteract these consequences and avoid negative health outcomes. DTCA may also suggest that cancer and disease is quite common among the population, feeding a sense of fatalism. People may believe that cancer and other diseases are inevitable, and therefore preventative behaviors that may be difficult or seem to involve deprivation from pleasurable activities may not be considered worth the effort.

The concept of exposure is critical to considering the potential effects of DTCA on cancer prevention. Communication is central to promoting critical health behaviors that can prevent cancer [12]. As much as 50-65% of cancer is the result of behavior thereby potentially preventable [1]. A substantial body of research has shown that deliberate public health communication campaigns can have a favorable effect leading to behavioral choices that prevent cancer and reduce its incidence [13]. But, the success of a public health communication campaign depends on the degree to which it can generate exposure to its messages [14]. The more exposure a campaign can produce the greater its effects on the target behavior. The amount of exposure that pharmaceutical companies have been generating with broadcast advertising is perhaps unprecedented in the history of deliberate campaigns targeting health behavior. The meta-message of DTCA that pharmaceutical products will solve all health problems, stands in stark contrast to the message that lifestyle change can prevent cancer. Theoretical models of health behavior change, which have guided and driven health communication campaigns, suggest that beliefs resulting from DTCA exposure could be associated with less behavior that could prevent cancer [15]. This leads to the hypothesis that repeated exposure to the meta-message of DTCA results in: (1) stronger perceptions and beliefs that pharmaceutical products and healthcare services will solve all health problems, including cancer; and (2) weaker perceptions and beliefs that lifestyle change and behavioral choices are important in preventing cancer and other health problems. The meta-message of DTCA may render public health campaigns aimed at increasing behavior to prevent cancer less effective. A recent IOM report noted that nearly half of all American adults have low health literacy that compromises their ability to understand and act on health information [16]. These individuals may be particularly vulnerable to the meta-message of DTCA, potentially making attempts to reduce cancer disparities more difficult.

The US is the only country besides New Zealand that allows DTCA for prescription drugs. If we assume that DTCA is here to stay we need to maximize the public health benefit and limit potential adverse public health effects. There is an urgent need for research addressing this hypothesis so that policy regulating DTCA can take a more comprehensive view.

Acknowledgement

Supported by the Robert Wood Johnson Health and Society Scholars Program

References

[1] Lerman, C., B. Rimer, and T. Glynn, Priorities in behavioral research in cancer prevention and control. Prev Med, 1997. 26(5 Pt 2): p. S3-9.

[2] Lyles, A., Direct marketing of pharmaceuticals to consumers. Annu Rev Public Health, 2002. 23: p. 73-91.

[3] Perri, M., 3rd, S. Shinde, and R. Banavali, The past, present, and future of direct-to-consumer prescription drug advertising. Clin Ther, 1999. 21(10): p. 1798-811; discussion 1797.

[4] Rosenthal, M.B., et al., Promotion of prescription drugs to consumers. N Engl J Med, 2002. 346(7): p. 498-505.

[5] Kravitz, R.L., Direct-to-consumer advertising of prescription drugs. West J Med, 2000. 173(4): p. 221-2.

[6] Lancet, Europe on the brink of direct-to-consumer drug advertising. Lancet, 2002. 359(9319): p. 1709.

[7] Findlay, S.D., Direct-to-consumer promotion of prescription drugs. Economic implications for patients, payers and providers. Pharmacoeconomics, 2001. 19(2): p. 109-19.

[8] Mintzes, B., et al., How does direct-to-consumer advertising (DTCA) affect prescribing? A survey in primary care environments with and without legal DTCA. Cmaj, 2003. 169(5): p. 405-12.

[9] Mintzes, B., For and against: Direct to consumer advertising is medicalising normal human experience: For. Bmj, 2002. 324(7342): p. 908-9.

[10] Hollon, M.F., Direct-to-consumer marketing of prescription drugs: creating consumer demand. Jama, 1999. 281(4): p. 382-4.

[11] Woloshin, S., Schwartz, L.M., Welch H.G., The value of benefit data in direct-to-consumer drug ads. Health Affairs, 2004. Web Exclusive(W4): p. 234-245.

[12] Kreps, G.J., The impact of communication on cancer risk, incidence, morbidity, mortality, and quality of life. Health Commun, 2003. 15(2): p. 161-9.

[13] Kreps, G.L., Chapelsky Massimilla, D., Cancer communications research and health outcomes: Review and challenge. Communication Studies, 2002. 53(4): p. 318-336.

[14] Hornik, R.C., Public health communication: Evidence for behavior change. 2002, Mahwah, NJ: L. Erlbaum Associates.

[15] Fishbein, M., The role of theory in HIV prevention. AIDS Care, 2000. 12(3):p. 273-8. IOM, Health literacy: A prescription to end confusion. 2004, Washington, D.C.: National Academy of Sciences.

In: Cancer Prevention Research Trends
Editors: Louis Braun and Maximilian Lange

ISBN: 978-1-60456-639-0
© 2008 Nova Science Publishers, Inc.

Chapter II

Gastric, Colorectal and Pancreatic Carcinoma: The Relationship between Hemostasis and Cancer Prognostic Markers

Hussain Alizadeh, [*] *Shaikhah Al-Tajer,* [†] *and Shaker A. Mousa* [‡]

[*]University of Pecs, Faculty of General Medicine, 1st Department of Internal Medicine, 13-Ifjusag Street, 7624-Pecs, Hungary
[†]AlAin Medical District, Tawam Hospital, Department of Medicine, PO Box 15258, AlAin, AbuDhabi, United Arab Emirates and
[‡]Pharmaceutical Research Institute at Albany and Albany College of Pharmacy, 106 New Scotland Avenue, Albany, NY 12208-3492, USA

Abstract

Patients with different types of nonhematological, solid organ tumor (esophageal adenocarcinoma, gastric cancer, colorectal cancer, exocrine pancreatic adenocarcinoma, or adenocarcinoma of gallbladder) were studied. Detailed monitoring upon admission and prior to any cancer-related intervention and on a weekly basis post-intervention (chemotherapy, radiation or surgery) but not anticoagulant for up to 18 weeks were carried out. Natural inhibitors of coagulation (protein C, protein S, and antithrombin), and D-dimer and prothrombin activation peptide F1+2 as markers of the status of fibrinolytic and coagulation systems were determined. In all cases the levels of hypercoagulable markers were elevated directly correlated with tumor markers and radiological findings. Additionally, the level of naturally occurring coagulation inhibitors all decreased with tumor progression. Thus, determination of hemostasis activation state can be used to assess the tumor prognosis, and early anticoagulation prophylaxis might prevent venous thromboembolism and impair tumor progression.

KeyWords: hemostasis, cancer, tumor markers, computed tomographic imaging, prognosis, diagnosis

Introduction

Thromboembolic events are a well-recognized complication of malignant disease and can contribute significantly to the morbidity and mortality of this disease [1–4]. Although the close relationship between tumor growth and the activation of blood coagulation has been known since 1865, when Professor Armand Trousseau first described the clinical association between primary or idiopathic venous thromboembolism (VTE) and occult malignancy, it is only in the last 2 or 3 decades that significant advances in this field have been achieved.

It is now well known that the clinical manifestation of thrombosis in the malignant disease can be very different and vary from localized VTE to disseminated intravascular coagulation (DIC). In addition, a subclinical activation of blood coagulation or "hypercoagulable state" is present in almost all cancer patients, even without symptoms of thrombosis. Thrombosis in the setting of malignancy portends aggressive disease, increased metastasis, and an overall poorer prognosis [5]. There is a 20-50% incidence of thrombosis in patients with metastatic cancer who have undergone postmortem examinations [6].

A number of pathogenetic factors have been identified showing that activation of coagulation in cancer is a complex phenomenon involving many different pathways of the hemostatic system and numerous interactions of the tumor cell with other blood cells, including platelets, monocytes and endothelial cells.

Even more recently, prospective clinical trials have definitely demonstrated that patients with idiopathic VTE are at significantly higher risk for a subsequent diagnosis of malignancy as compared to patients with secondary VTE (i.e., VTE due to known causes, such as congenital thrombophilia, the use of oral contraceptives, pregnancy and immobilization, among others). This risk is significantly increased by anti-tumor interventions, including surgery and chemotherapy.

Neoplastic cells can activate the clotting system directly, thereby generating thrombin, or indirectly, by stimulating mononuclear cells to synthesize and express various procoagulants [7–9]. Cancer cells and chemotherapeutic agents can injure endothelial cells and thereby intensify the hyper-coagulability [10–12].

The procoagulant state in cancer arises mostly from the capacity of tumor cells to express and release substances with procoagulant activities. Tissue factor (TF) and cancer procoagulant (CP) are two procoagulant activities that have been described and well documented in cancer patients [13–16]. Consistent with the shift of the hemostasis balance toward hypercoagulation in cancer, several studies have shown reduced levels of inhibitors of coagulation such as protein C (PC), protein S (PS), and antithrombin (AT) in cancer patients. These decreased levels of inhibitors might result from an increased consumption as a consequence of the activation of coagulation or from a defective hepatic synthesis or both mechanisms combined [17]. Chemotherapy and hormonal treatment can also induce an acquired deficiency in inhibitors [18, 19]. Different sensitive assays to assess the hypercoagulant state have been developed and applied to cancer studies [20, 21]. Among them are fibrinopeptide A (FPA), prothrombin activation peptide fragment 1+2 (F1+2), D-dimers, thrombin-antithrombin (TAT), plasmin-antiplasmin (PAP), decreased AT, PC and PS. There are commercially available immunoenzymatic assays or radioimmunoassay for the determination of these parameters [20–22]. In this investigation, we evaluated the changes in hemostatic parameters and their relation to cancer prognosis.

Aim of the Study

The study was primarily designed to determine whether hemostatic parameters were correlated with changes in imaging findings, tumor stage, and characteristic tumor markers changes. The tumor markers which were used in this study are recommended in follow up of patients with different types of solid tumor. These tumor markers are not tumor-specific, but they might be used as a useful tool for both diagnosis and follow up of these patients and also to assess the efficacy of the treatment. The prespecified criteria for evaluation were usefulness of these hypercoagulability markers in the follow up of this group of patients and also their use as reliable cancer prognostic markers.

Materials and Methods

Selection of Patients

Patients were eligible for enrollment in the study if they were over the age of 16 years and they had been diagnosed as having solid organ cancer. The patients were enrolled in this study prior to any type of treatment. Additional criteria for enrollment were absence of previous thromboembolic event in the past 12 months, absence of any heparin derivatives, oral anticoagulant agents and also antiplatelet drugs. Patients with suspected distant metastasis were excluded. Patients who received any type of anticoagulant or hormonal treatment in the past 6 months were also excluded. Patients having abnormal kidney and liver function tests were also not enrolled.

Baseline Characteristics of the Patients

A total of 32 patients were enrolled in the study over a period of 18 months, but 2 patients were excluded from the final evaluation of study because of the development of thromboembolic events during the period of study. The baseline characteristics of the eligible patients are summarized in Table 1. A summary of tumor types, treatment schedules, and chemotherapeutic regimens that were used (all standard internationally recommended protocols) are listed in Tables 2 and 3.

Table 1. Baseline Characteristics of Eligible Patients

Age (yr)	
Median	54
Range	26-72
ECOG performance score	0–1
Average no. chemotherapy cycles	8
Female	2
Male	1

Table 1. (Continued)

Smoking	
Female	2
Male	14
Alcohol intake	
Female	0
Male	4
Other malignancy	
Female	1
Male	0

Table 2. Summary of Tumor Types and Treatment

Tumor Type and Stage	*Treatment*
Colorectal adenocarcinoma, tubulovillous adenoma, Dukes B2 stage (16 males)	Surgical resection followed by adjuvant chemotherapy
Pancreatic adenocarcinoma, stage III (2 females, 2 males)	Surgical resection followed by systemic chemotherapy and radiotherapy
Esophageal adenocarcinoma, stage IIB (2 males)	Primary systemic chemotherapy and radiation followed by surgical resection (esophagectomy)
Gallbladder adenocarcinoma, stage II (1 male, 1 female)	Surgical resection followed by chemotherapy and local radiotherapy
Gastric adenocarcinoma, stage II (6 males)	Surgical resection (together with lymphadenectomy) followed by chemotherapy and radiation therapy

Table 3. Chemotherapeutic Regimens Used

Tumor Type	*Regimen Used*
Colorectal adenocarcinoma	5 FU + folinic acid for 8–12 cycles every 2–4 weeks
Gastric adenocarcinoma	Mainly 5 FU + folinic acid + cisplatin *or* ECF, but ELF also used occasionally again every 3–4 weeks and for at least 6–8 courses (depending on the response)
Esophageal adenocarcinoma	Cisplatin + 5 FU every 3–4 weeks prior to surgery and irradiation for 2–3 cycles and after surgery to repeat the same regimen for 2–3 additional cycles; ECF protocol also used in 1 case
Pancreatic adenocarcinoma	5 FU + folinic acid every 4 weeks for at least 6 cycles with radiation therapy

ECF = epirubin + cisplatin + 5 FU; ELF = etoposide + folinic acid + 5 FU; 5 FU = 5 fluorouracil.

Plasma levels of D-dimer, F1+2, AT, PC, and PS activity were measured at the onset of diagnosis, pre- and post-surgery, and after the completion of each chemotherapy course. Their levels were correlated with the levels of tumor markers. Baseline values of those markers in age-matched healthy subjects are shown in Table 4.

Table 4: Normal Ranges for the Various Hemostatic Parameters in Age-Matched Subjects

Hemostatic Parameters	Normal Reference Values
Antithrombin activity	Ref. range: 65–140%
Protein C activity	Ref. range: 70–140%
Free protein S antigen	Ref. range: 65–140%
Protein S activity	Ref. range: 60–140%
D-dimer	Ref. range: 0.0–0.3 mg/l
Prothrombin fragment 1+2	Ref. range: 0.32–1.1 nmol/l

Each sample was tested for AT activity using thrombin (AT-IIa) as the substrate; PC activity, using both clotting (PC-Cl) and chromogenic (PC-Chr) methods; PS activity; D-dimer; and F1+2 using immunoassays, ELISA, clotting, and chromogenic methods [23–28]. The reagents and kits used for these different assays were obtained from Dade Behring, Inc. (Deerfield, IL), Stago International (Parsippany, NJ), and R&D Systems, Inc. (Minneapolis, MN).

The imaging techniques that were used for diagnosis and staging were based on international recommendations for each disease category. These findings were reviewed by 2 different radiologists.

Study Design

Patients were stratified according to ECOG (Zubrod) performance status score, and those with ECOG score of 0-1 were enrolled in the study. Baseline AT, PS, PC, D-dimer and prothrombin activation peptide F1+2 as hemostatic parameters and characteristic tumor markers according to the type of tumor were measured [20–22]. Staging of cancer at various anatomic sites was done as developed by the American Joint Committee on Cancer (AJCC) in cooperation with the TNM Committee of the International Union Against Cancer (UICC). The International Histological Classification of Tumours provided by the World Health Organization (WHO) was used for pathologic classification and definition of tumor types. Physical examination, imaging, endoscopy, biopsy, and surgical exploration were used for clinical classification and staging. Histologic grading was also used for qualitative assessment of the differentiation of the tumors. All the patients were treated according to the internationally recommended therapeutic regimens, and they were closely followed up to evaluate the state of their malignant disease. The hemostatic parameters, the tumor marker and the imaging techniques were repeated after the completion of 2 full chemotherapeutic regimens. In those cases where surgical intervention was indicated prior to the start of chemotherapy, the coagulation parameters and tumor markers were measured prior to the surgery and the hemostatic values were repeated after the end of surgery. None of these patients were on any kind of medications which would interfere with the results of coagulation studies. During each visit physical examination, vital signs and medication history were taken and any changes in these findings were registered. If the patient developed febrile neutropenia as a complication of a chemotherapeutic agent, the hemostatic parameters were measured at the onset of the diagnosis of febrile neutropenia and thereafter.

Statistical Analysis

Statistical analysis was performed by two-way analysis of variance (ANOVA) comparing markers of hemostasis activation at admission to post-admission for each subject and with respect to average control values; differences were considered significant at $p < 0.05$ or less.

Results

Gastric Carcinoma (Stage II and IIIA)

Prothrombin F1+2 and D-dimer levels increased over time post-treatment in 4 of 5 gastric adenocarcinoma patients, with a peak increase at weeks 8–11 (Figure 1A, 1B). In 1 of the 5, the levels of F1+2 and D-dimer were normalized (Figure 1A, 1B). In contrast, the natural anticoagulants PC-activity, PS-activity, and AT-activity levels showed progressive decrease in 4 of 5 patients, with a peak decrease at 8–11 weeks (Figures 1C–1E). In 1 of the 5 patients, the levels of those natural anticoagulants were normalized (Figure 1C–1E).

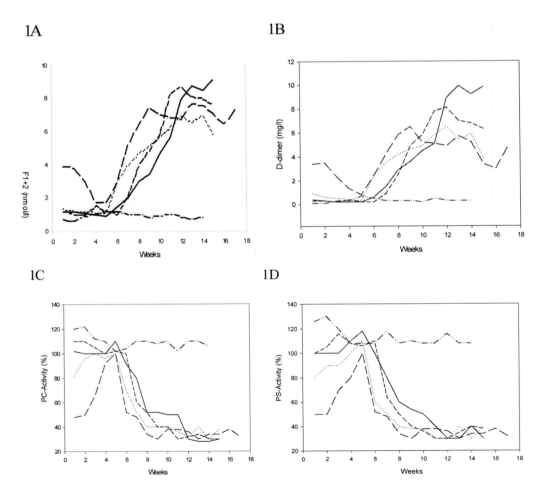

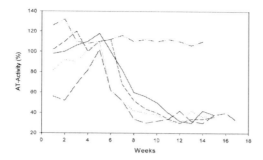

Figure 1. Hemostatic activation markers at admission or at initial presentation or at time of diagnosis (week 1) and post-treatment on a weekly basis for up to 18 weeks in gastric adenocarcinoma (stage II/IIIa) patients (n = 5). Figure 1A: F1+2 (nmol/L), and 1B: D-dimer (mg/L). Natural anticoagulant markers at admission or at initial presentation or at time of diagnosis (week 1) and post-treatment on a weekly basis for up to 18 weeks. Figure 1C: PC activity (%), Figure 1D: PS activity (%), and Figure 1E: AT activity (%). Four out of five patients showed significant (p <0.01) increase in F1+2 and D-dimer (Figure 1A, B). In contrast, in those 4 out of 5 subjects, significant (p <0.01) decline in natural anticoagulants was shown (Figure 1C–1E).

Colorectal Adenocarcinoma in Male Patients (Dukes B2 Stage)

Plasma levels of F1+2 and D-dimer showed highest level at admission, with a significant decline post-treatment. About 50% of the patients (6 of 12) started with normal ranges of F1+2 and D-dimer, and the remainder showed 100% response post-treatment, with normalized levels of both markers by weeks 6–10, depending on the starting deficit (Figure 2A, 2B). In contrast, the natural anticoagulants demonstrated the reverse trend to that of F1+2 and D-dimer (Figures 2C–2E). About 50% of the patients showed significantly lower levels at admission, with 100% response to treatment and full normalization by week 6 (Figures 2C–2E).

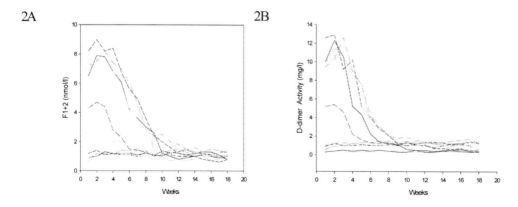

Figure 2. (Continued)

2C   2D

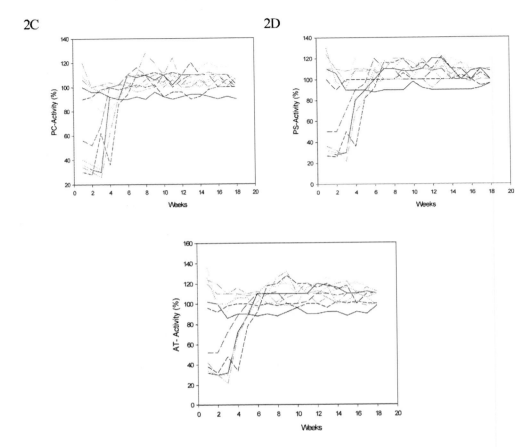

Figure 2. Hemostatic activation markers at admission or at initial presentation or at time of diagnosis (week 1) and post-treatment on a weekly basis for up to 18 weeks in colorectal adenocarcinoma in male patients (Dukes B2 stage). Figure 2A: F1+2 (nmol/L), and 2B: D-dimer (mg/L). Natural anticoagulant markers at admission or at initial presentation or at time of diagnosis (week 1) and post-treatment on a weekly basis for up to 18 weeks. Figure 2C: PC activity (%), Figure 2D: PS activity (%), and Figure 2E: AT activity (%). At admission, 50% of patients showed significant (p <0.05) elevations in F1+2/D-dimer and significant decline (p <0.05) of natural anticoagulants. All patients showed significant normalization in F1+2, D-dimer as well as natural anticoagulants by week 10.

Pancreatic Adenocarcinoma (Stage III)

A progressive increase in F1+2 and D-dimer in 3 of 4 patients post-treatment was shown (Figure 3A, 3B). In 1 of 4, a decline in both F1+2 and D-dimer was shown up to the first 12 weeks post-treatment, followed by rapid increase that caught up with other cases (Figure 3A, 3B). In contrast, the natural anticoagulants (PC, PS, and AT activities) demonstrated the reverse trend to that of F1+2 and D-dimer (Figures 3C–3E). Most of the patients (3 of 4) showed no response to treatment and full normalization in 1 of the 4 by week 7 but followed by rapid decline by weeks 12–14 (Figures 3C–3E).

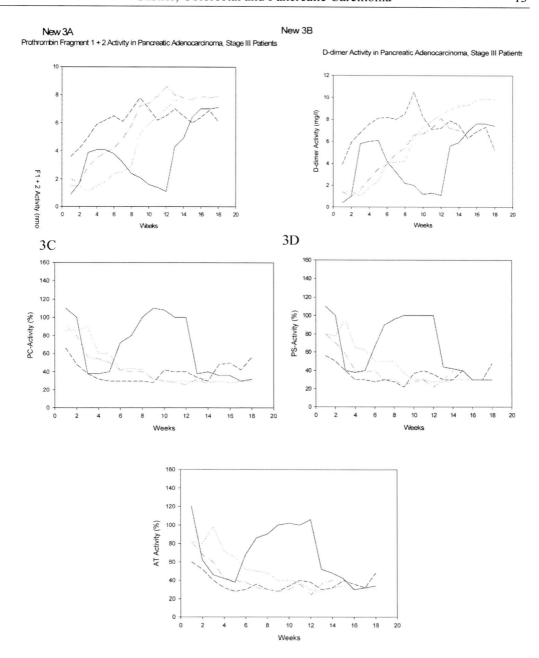

Figure 3. Hemostatic activation markers at admission or at initial presentation or at time of diagnosis (week 1) and post-treatment on a weekly basis for up to 18 weeks in pancreatic adenocarcinoma patients (stage III). Figure 3A: Prothrombin Fragment 1+2 (nmol/L) activity, and 3B: D-dimer (mg/L). Natural anticoagulant markers at admission or at initial presentation or at time of diagnosis (week 1) and post-treatment on a weekly basis for up to 18 weeks. Figure 3C: PC activity (%), Figure 3D: PS activity (%), and Figure 3E: AT activity (%). A significantly (p <0.05) progressive increase in F1+2 and D-dimer in 3 of 4 patients was shown. The other subject showed initial decline, but levels approached those other 3 subjects by week 15–18.

Tumor Marker (CEA) in Colorectal Cancer Patients

Different levels of elevation (20–300 ug/L) above normal ranges were shown at admission (Figure 4). A 100% response to treatment in the reversal of elevated levels of CEA by weeks 5-10 depending on the initial levels were shown (Figure 4). Patients with highest levels of CEA at admission showed the highest F1+2/D-dimer and the highest deficit in natural anticoagulants.

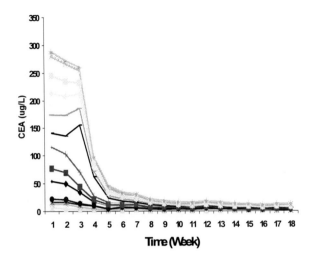

Figure 4. Tumor marker (CEA, ug/L) at admission or at initial presentation or at time of diagnosis (week 1) and post-treatment on a weekly basis for up to 18 weeks in colorectal carcinoma in female patients. All patients showed variable levels of elevations in CEA, with normalization post-treatment by week 5–10.

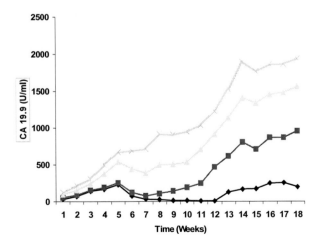

Figure 5. Tumor marker (CA 19.9, U/ml) at admission or at initial presentation or at time of diagnosis (week 1) and post-treatment on a weekly basis for up to 18 weeks in pancreatic cancer patients. A significant ($p < 0.01$) progressive increase in CA was shown. Variable levels of increase in CA were shown among the different subjects.

Tumor Marker (CA 19.9) in Pancreatic Cancer Patients

Different levels of progressive elevation above normal ranges were shown post-treatment (Figure 5). An excellent response to treatment was shown in 1 of 4 patients (Figure 5). Patients with highest levels of CA 19.9 showed the highest F1+2/D-dimer and the highest deficit in natural anticoagulants.

CT Imaging

Pancreatic cancer patients with highest tumor marker (CA19.9), highest F1+2 or D-dimer, and lowest natural anticoagulants (PC, PS, AT activities) showed the largest tumor mass. A representative CT imaging of a patient with a relatively large tumor mass at admission is shown in Figure 6A. This patient showed a good response to treatment (week 8), as shown in Figure 6B. This patient showed the lowest CA19.9 levels, as well as a normalized level of F1+2/D-dimer and PC/PS/AT activities at week 8.

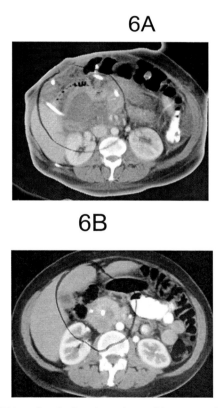

Figure 6. (A) At diagnosis—CT imaging in female patient with pancreatic adenocarcinoma, large tumor mass, with highly elevated tumor marker CA19.9 and hemostatic markers. (B) Post-treatment—CT imaging in female patient with pancreatic adenocarcinoma who showed reduction in tumor mass and the tumor marker CA 19.9. Improvements in hemostatic markers are shown as well.

CT Imaging in Gastric Adenocarcinoma Patients

An excellent trend between tumor mass and hemostasis activation was also shown. A representative case of preoperative CT in a male patient with stage II/IIIa showed the existence of a large obstructive tumor blocking the gastric lumen and infiltrating the stomach wall (Figure 7A). Early elevation in hemostasis activation markers was also shown. In Figure 7B, CT imaging after surgery and chemotherapy illustrates the excellent response and the normalization of hemostasis markers.

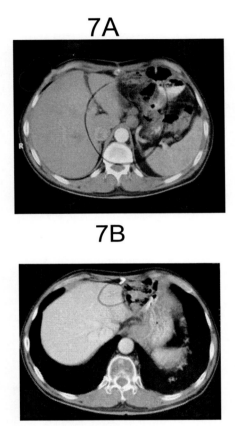

Figure 7. (A) At diagnosis—CT preoperative imaging in male patient with stage II/IIIa gastric adenocarcinoma. The tumor as shown is obstructing the gastric lumen and infiltrating the wall of the stomach. Early changes in hemostatic activity markers were shown. (B) After surgery—CT imaging postoperative adjuvant chemotherapy, showing excellent response. Hemostatic markers remained close to normal ranges.

CT Imaging in a Female Patient with Dukes Stage B2 Colon Adenocarcinoma

This illustrates a large obstructive tumor mass (Figure 8A) that was also seen with colonoscopy. At 4 weeks post-surgery followed by chemotherapy, no tumor was detected (Figure 8B). Normalization of tumor marker and hemostasis marker levels was also demonstrated at 4–18 weeks.

8A

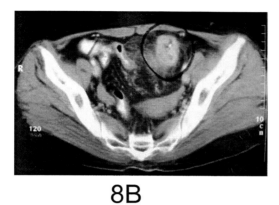

8B

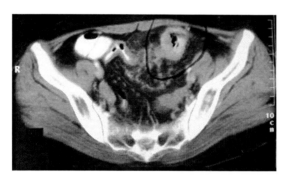

Figure 8. (A) Representative CT image in woman with Dukes stage B2 colon adenocarcinoma (tubular) preoperative, showing large obstructive tumor. Elevated levels of tumor markers and hemostasis activation markers were documented at admission. (B) Representative CT image at 4 weeks post-surgery showing successful removal of tumor, which coincides with normalization of tumor markers and hemostasis markers.

Discussion

The interaction between components of the hemostatic system and cancer cells are multifactorial. Strong clinical evidences are accumulating on the prothrombotic or hypercoagulable tendency of cancer patients, which is enhanced by any type of anticancer treatment, such as chemotherapy or surgery [8]. The interactive mechanisms between coagulation system and malignancy include some general responses of the host to the tumor cells (angiogenesis, inflammation, acute phase, etc.) and the specific interaction of tumor cells with the blood elements, mainly platelets and leukocytes, with hemostatic systems, including fibrinolysis and clotting components and also with vascular endothelial cells [7, 29, 30]. It is difficult at present to identify the relative weight of these interactions on the basis of the well-recognized clinical evidence of hypercoagulable status in tumor patients.

Our prospective study was designed to evaluate the changes in clotting parameters in patients with solid tumors and to examine their correlation with tumor stage, imaging findings and also with changes in characteristic tumor markers. In this study we mainly focused on specific abnormalities of hemostasis in these groups of patients. Inclusion in the study required tissue diagnosis for histopathologic classification, detailed imaging techniques for exact staging, and absence of any medications that might interfere with the results of hypercoagulation markers. The study design and outcomes evaluations mirrored those used in prior studies, except that our study used more than one coagulation parameter for a more detailed assessment of the changes in hemostatic system in cancer patients.

Except for a slight difference in the gender ratio, the analysis of patients who met the prespecified criteria for evaluation showed that the hypercoagulable parameters were directly correlated with tumor progression and rise in characteristic tumor markers. It is a well known fact that the tumor cells produce and express different procoagulant substances (such as TF, CP, and plasminogen activators), and these factors interact with the vascular cells, blood cells, coagulation system and fibrinolytic system, and will lead to a disturbance in the normal hemostasis, which finally will result in an abnormal hypercoagulable status. We studied the prognostic values of F1+2, D-dimer, and natural inhibitors of abnormal coagulation in patients with solid tumors, but so far no convincing data have allowed identification of one of these hypercoagulability markers as a reliable disease prognostic marker [31].

Parallel with the hemostatic parameters, the characteristic tumor markers were also measured. In all studied cases, there was a direct correlation among changes in the hemostatic parameters, tumor markers and radiological imaging findings (e.g., rise in D-dimer, F1+2 was associated with a drop in AT, PS, PC, which was directly correlated with a rise in tumor markers and a progression of the malignant diseases in imaging findings).

The relationship between the hypercoagulable state and the tumor progression and the occurrence of metastasis has not been well established. Larger studies on tests that could have a reliable predictive value in tumor progression are needed. Much more information is needed, and only large-scale clinical trials will unequivocally establish whether these hypercoagulable parameters have strong predictive values and whether the modulation of the hemostatic system will modify the process of tumor progression and metastatic dissemination.

References

[1]   Billroth T. *Lectures on Surgical Pathology and Therapeutics: A Handbook for Students and Practitioners*. 8th ed. (translated). London, The New Sydenham Society; 1878.

[2]   Dvorak HF. Abnormalities of hemostasis in malignant disease. In Colman RW, Hirsh J, Marder VJ, Salzman EW, eds. *Hemostasis and Thrombosis: Basic Principles and Clinical Practice*. Philadelphia, Lippincott; 1994, 1238–1254.

[3]   Sporul EE. Carcinoma and venous thrombosis: the frequency of association of carcinoma in the body or tail of the pancreas with multiple venous thrombosis. *Am J Cancer* 1938, 34, 566-585.

[4]   Trousseau A. Phlegmasia alba dolens. In *Clinique medicale de l'Hotel-Dieu de Paris*. vol. 3. Paris, Bailliere, 1865, 654-712.

[5]   Sorensen HT, Mellemjkaer L, Olsen JH, Baron JA. Prognosis of cancers associated with venous thromboembolism. *N Engl J Med* 2000, 343, 1846-1850.

[6]   Slichter SJ, Harker LA. Hemostasis in malignancy. *Ann N Y Acad Sci* 1974, 230, 252-261.

[7]   Falanga A, Barbui T, Rickles FR, Levine MN. Guidelines for clotting studies in cancer patients. *Thromb Haemost* 1993, 70, 540-542.

[8]   Falanga A, Ofosu FA, Delaini F, Oldani E, Dewar L, Lui L, et al. The hypercoagulable state in cancer patients: evidence for impaired thrombin inhibition. *Blood Coagul Fibrinolysis* 1994, 5(suppl), S19-S23.

[9]   Mousa SA. Anticoagulants in thrombosis and cancer: the missing link. *Semin Thromb Hemost* 2002, 28, 45-52.

[10]   Celi A, Lorenzet R, Furie B, Furie BC. Platelet-leukocyte-endothelial cell interaction on the blood vessel wall. *Semin Hematol* 1997, 34, 327-335.

[11]   Napoleone M, Di Santo A, Lorenzet R. Monocytes upregulate endothelial cell expression of tissue factor: a role for cell-cell contact and cross-talk. *Blood* 1997, 89, 541-549.

[12]   Semeraro N, Colucci M. Tissue factor in health and disease. *Thromb Haemost* 1997, 78, 759-764.

[13]   Edwards RL, Silver J, Rickles FR. Human tumor procoagulants: registry of the Subcommittee on Haemostasis and Malignancy of the Scientific and Standardization Committee, International Society on Thrombosis and Haemostasis. *Thromb Haemost* 1993, 69, 205-213.

[14]   Gordon SG, Cross BA. A factor X activating cysteine protease from malignant tissue. *J Clin Invest* 1981, 67, 1665.

[15]   Gordon SG, Mielicki WP. Cancer procoagulant—a factor X activator, tumor marker and growth factor from malignant tissue. *Blood Coagul Fibrinolysis* 1997, 6/2, 73-86.

[16]   Rao LVM. Tissue factor as a tumor procoagulant. *Cancer Metastasis Rev* 1992, 11, 249-266.

[17]   Rickles FR, Levine M, Edwards RL. Hemostatic alteration in cancer patients. *Cancer Metastasis Rev* 1992, 11, 237-248.

[18]   Conard J, Horellou MH, Van Dreden P, Potevin F, Zittoun R, Samama M. Decrease in protein C in L-asparaginase-treated patients. *Br J Haematol* 1985, 59, 725-727.

[19]   Lee AYY, Levine MN. The thrombophilic state induced by therapeutic agents in the cancer patients. *Semin Thromb Hemost* 1999, 25/2, 137-146.

[20]   Manucci PM. Markers of hypercoagulability in cancer patients. *Haemostasis* 1997, 27(suppl 1), 25-31.

[21]   Tripodi A, Manucci PM. Markers of activated coagulation and their usefulness in the clinical laboratory. *Clin Chem* 1996, 2, 664-669.

[22]   Green K, Silverstein RL. Hypercoagulability in cancer. *Hematol Oncol Clin North Am* 1996, 10, 499-530.

[23]   Sallah S, Husain A, Sigounas V, Wan J, Turturro F, Sigounas G, et al. Plasma coagulation markers in patients with solid tumors and venous thromboembolic disease receiving oral anticoagulation therapy. *Clin Cancer Res* 2004, 10, 7238-7243.

[24] Caine GJ, Lip GY, Stonelake PS, Ryan P, Blann AD. Platelet activation, coagulation and angiogenesis in breast and prostate carcinoma. *Thromb Haemost* 2004, 2, 185-190.

[25] Unsal E, Atalay F, Atikcan S, Yilmaz A. Prognostic significance of hemostatic parameters in patients with lung cancer. *Respir Med* 2004, 98, 93-98.

[26] Lind SE, Caprini JA, Goldshteyn S, Dohnal JC, Vesely SK, Shevrin DH. Correlates of thrombin generation in patients with advanced prostate cancer. *Thromb Haemost* 2003, 89, 185-189.

[27] Roselli M, Mineo TC, Basili S, Mariotti S, Martini F, Bellotti A, et al. Vascular endothelial growth factor (VEGF-A) plasma levels in non-small cell lung cancer: relationship with coagulation and platelet activation markers. *Thromb Haemost* 2003, 89, 177-184.

[28] Bozic M, Blinc A, Stegnar M. D-dimer, other markers of haemostasis activation and soluble adhesion molecules in patients with different clinical probabilities of deep vein thrombosis. *Thromb Res* 2002, 108, 107-114.

[29] Donati MB, Poggi A. Malignancy and haemostasis. *Br J Haematol* 1980, 44, 173-182.

[30] Falanga A, Rickles FR. Pathophysiology of the thrombophilic state in cancer patients. *Semin Thromb Hemost* 1999, 25, 173-182.

[31] Gouin-Thibault I, Samama MM. Laboratory diagnosis of the thrombophilic state in cancer patients. *Semin Thromb Hemost* 1999, 25/2, 167-172.

In: Cancer Prevention Research Trends
Editors: Louis Braun and Maximilian Lange

ISBN: 978-1-60456-639-0
© 2008 Nova Science Publishers, Inc.

Chapter III

Vitamin D Use among Older Adults in U.S.: Results from National Surveys 1997 To 2002

Euni Lee[1]*, Mary Maneno[1], Anthony K. Wutoh[1] and Seok-Woo Lee[2]

[1]Department of Clinical and Administrative Pharmacy Sciences, School of Pharmacy, Howard University, Washington, District of Columbia
[2]Division of Periodontics, School of Dental and Oral Surgery, Columbia University, New York, New York

Abstract

Osteoporosis is the most common bone disease leading to increased fracture risk and is associated with permanent disability and poor outcomes. Established guidelines emphasize the role of calcium/vitamin D supplementation for optimal management of osteoporosis. Current literature indicates under-diagnosis with osteoporosis, and under-use of anti-osteoporosis medications with calcium/vitamin D supplementation upon diagnosis. Few studies have evaluated utilization patterns and trends of vitamin D among the older US population for prevention and/or treatment, and even fewer studies have assessed the prevalence of vitamin D use evaluating national level databases. Therefore, this study was conducted to evaluate recent trends in vitamin D prescribing using two national databases; the National Ambulatory Medical Care Survey (NAMCS) and Medical Expenditure Panel Survey (MEPS) from 1997 to 2002. NAMCS is an annual survey conducted by the National Center for Health Statistics (NCHS). The Agency for Healthcare Research and Quality (AHRQ) conducts MEPS in conjunction with the NCHS. NAMCS and MEPS are important resources designed to provide information about health care use and costs (MEPS only) in the U.S. as indicated by visits made by non-institutionalized patients and individuals drawn from a nationally representative sub-sample of households across the nation. This study provides 6-year trends in vitamin D use, characteristics of individuals that are associated with vitamin D, and predictors of vitamin D prescribing. Our findings indicated that very few visits made by patients were

* Corresponding author:Euni Lee, Pharm.D, Ph.D. School of Pharmacy, Howard University 2300 Fourth Street NW, Washington, DC 20059. Telephone: (202) 806-4919; Fax: (202) 806-4478; E-mail: eunlee@howard.edu

associated with vitamin D prescriptions. The overall utilization of vitamin D therapy in the U.S. between1997 and 2002 was suboptimal. Older and female patients, and patients with an osteoporosis diagnosis were more likely to be receiving vitamin D therapy. Our findings support the need for greater awareness regarding vitamin D supplementation among patients who are 40 years and older, especially among male patients, through patient counseling. A coordinated effort and comprehensive programmatic approach among health care professional including physicians, dentists, nurses, pharmacists, and nutritionists are recommended to improve osteoporosis prevention and treatment.

Osteoporosis, a risk factor for fragility facture, is the most common bone disease in the U.S., affecting 44 million Americans.[1,2] Most fractures can lead to permanent disability with severe pain or even death [3,4,5], and unfortunately they often serve as the first clinical manifestation of disease.[5] Fragility fractures create a heavy economic burden. The national direct cost for osteoporotic hip fractures has been estimated at $18 billion (2002 dollars), and costs are continuing to rise.[1]

As part of the natural aging process after the age of about 30, bones begin to break down faster than new bone can be formed.[6] Age-related osteoporosis often occurs after menopause among women.[7] Osteoporotic fractures or kyphosis in elderly women was previously viewed as an unavoidable consequence of aging. However, osteoporosis can now be prevented, diagnosed, and treated before occurrence of any fracture as researchers have developed a better understanding of pathophysiology and therapeutic options. According to recent guidelines on osteoporosis prevention, diagnosis, and therapy from the National Institutes of Health and American Association of Clinical Endocrinologists (AACE), optimization of bone health must occur throughout life with a balanced diet rich in calcium and vitamin D and regular physical activity.[7, 8] Therefore, prevention of osteoporosis becomes especially important due to lack of effective methods for restoring high quality bone to the osteoporotic skeleton. [9]

As a fat soluble vitamin, vitamin D plays a major fole in bone mineralization. It is a major transcriptional regulator of the bone proteins; type I collagen and osteocalcin.[10] Calcium and vitamin D intake modulates age-related increases in parathyroid hormone levels and bone resoprtion.[7] The suggested major role of vitamin D in bone is to provide the proper microenvironment for bone mineralization through stimulation of the intestinal absorption of calcium and phosphate.[10]

The effects of vitamin D and calcium on bone and osteoporosis prevention have been discussed extensively in the literature and their supplemental use for fracture reduction was acknowledged by current practice guidelines.[5, 7, 8] Additionally, these recommendations emphasize the role of calcium and vitamin D supplementation for optimal treatment of osteoporosis with any anti-osteoporosis therapy.[5, 8] According to the Physician's Guide from the National Osteoporosis Foundation, at least 1200 mg per day of calcium and 400 to 800 IU per day of vitamin D is recommended for all individuals.[5] The AACE guidelines stated that adequate calcium and vitamin D intake is fundamental to prevention and treatment programs for postmenopausal osteoporosis.[8]

There are several randomized controlled trials that have shown the efficacy of calcium and vitamin D supplementation to increase bone mineral density (BMD), and therefore reduce fracture risk and falls.[11-15] However, limited evidence is available to support independent effects of vitamin D on bone protective benefit, [15-18] as most clinical trials involved combined use with calcium.[7, 19] Despite the established benefits of calcium and/or vitamin D among the elderly, little is known of either the prevalence and sufficiency of combined vitamin D and calcium use [20] or vitamin D intake alone [21]. Given the lack of published studies exploring utilization patterns of vitamin D medications among the general older adult population in the U.S., this study was conducted to evaluate recent trends in vitamin D prescribing using two national-level databases. The study's objectives were to estimate the prevalence of overall vitamin D use, to evaluate patient characteristics between vitamin D users and non-users, and to assess predictive factors of vitamin D use among patient characteristics such as age, gender, race, insurance type, region, metropolitan status, physician specialties, and osteoporosis diagnosis.

Methodology

Study Design and Population

This study is primarily descriptive and only includes patients in ambulatory care settings, where primary care physicians play a major role in therapeutic decision-making. Therefore, patients who were hospitalized or institutionalized were not a part of the study population. We included patients or patient visit records made by men and women 40 years of age and older. The age criterion of 40 years or older was selected because osteoporosis is more prevalent among postmenopausal women and an age distribution of menopause ranges from age 40 to 58 years.[22] In order to compare vitamin D use by gender, we also used the same age criterion for male patients.

Data Source

In this study, we evaluated recent national patterns of vitamin D use, analyzing data from the 1997 to 2002 using two national survey data; the National Ambulatory Medical Care Survey (NAMCS) from the National Center for Health Statistics, and the Medical Expenditure Panel Survey (MEPS) from the Agency for Healthcare Research and Quality. The NAMCS, which began in 1973, is an annual survey conducted by the National Center for Health Statistics (NCHS) and is a population-based estimate of service utilization.[23] NAMCS collected data on the utilization of ambulatory medical care services provided by office-based physicians from office visits.[23] NAMCS data provides an important tool for tracking ambulatory care utilization by providing information regarding national trends, medication use or practice patterns among various types of providers in the U.S.[23]

The MEPS is a nationally representative survey used to provide information on health care use, health condition, associated medications, expenditures, sources of payment, and insurance coverage for the U.S. civilian non-institutionalized population sponsored by the Agency for Healthcare Research and Quality (AHRQ) and the National Center for Health Statistics (NCHS). The survey includes a Household Component (HC), Prescribed Medicine (PM) database, and Medical Conditions files. This public use file provides details regarding demographic information on each patient, household reported prescribed medicines, and medical conditions. The survey includes a nationally representative sample of the civilian non-institutionalized population of the U.S. The MEPS is a current data resource to capture the changing dynamics of the health care delivery and insurance system.[24]

One of the differences between NAMCS and MEPS is the unit of measurement; an office visit is the unit of measure from the NAMCS, and each individual patient is the unit of measure for MEPS. Office-based physicians provide data on patients' office visits including up to three diagnoses, types of counseling, and up to six medications per visit. In addition, NAMCS provides information on the physician specialty, type of practice, limited patient demographics, and types of payers or insurance.[23] NAMCS data are directly collected from participating physicians, thereby it provides information about physician's prescription behavior.

NAMCS uses a multistage probability sampling design, involving probability samples of primary sampling units (PSU), physician practices within the PSU, and patient visits within the sampled practices. Statistics derived from NAMCS data are representative of all ambulatory office visits to physicians engaged in office-based patient care.[23] The sample from 1997 and 1998 consisted of 24,715 and 23,339 completed patient visits, respectively.[23, 25] Each visit record is assigned an inflation factor called the "patient visit weight." By aggregating the visit weights provided by NCHS from the sample records, a national estimate of office visits can be obtained.[26, 27]

Definition of Vitamin D Products

A record was considered a vitamin D visit or a patient with a vitamin D prescription if one or more vitamin D products were identified from the database as being prescribed, provided, or continued by the physician. Vitamin D products include all single entity, or combination products with following drug entities; calcifediol, cholecalciferol, dihydrotachysterol, ergocalciferol, vitamin D, and calcitriol. All drugs that were prescribed, ordered, or provided to patients, or visits made by patients were listed from each database. Since drug related variables from NAMCS included a generic name field, generic names were used to identify vitamin D records. In the MEPS dataset, the drug name field contained both brand and generic names. Therefore, vitamin D products were identified from the Web-Lexicon[TM] Multum database (Multum Information Systems, Denver, CO, 2002) using both brand and generic names and they were matched to the drug names from MEPS data. Each vitamin D record from MEPS was validated by two pharmacists.

Statistical Methods

The analytic goal of this study focused on estimating the prevalence of vitamin D use for osteoporosis prevention and treatment, describing its use by patient characteristics, and evaluating predictive factors for vitamin D use. Two analytic files were created from the two databases by combining information from 1997 to 2002. In order to obtain national visit estimates, the assigned patient visit weights were aggregated. Both annual visit rates and overall prevalence were estimated and are reported by age group, racial category, insurance type, physician specialty, and location of the physician office by geographical region

(Northeast, Midwest, South, and West) as well as metropolitan (urban) vs. non-metropolitan (non-urban) location.

While all figures representing national estimates were based on weighted estimates, a few statistical analyses and the number of vitamin D users were based on the unweighted sample because national estimates based on relative standard errors higher than 30 percent are considered to be unreliable.[26, 27] Bivariate differences in the prevalence of vitamin D therapy by visit characteristics were tested using the χ^2 test and unadjusted odds ratios (OR) were calculated. Adjusted OR were calculated using a logistic regression model accounting for the complex sampling design, and the model included covariates such as race, age, metropolitan status, geographic region, and insurance type. All analyses were performed with SAS statistical software, version 9.1 (SAS Institute, Cary, NC).

Results

When patient visits from physician's office were evaluated using the 1997-2002 NAMCS data, the study population made an estimated number of 2,874 million visits. (Table 1) The mean age of the patients from NAMCS was 61.9 years (SD=13.7) and higher than that of MEPS. About 60% of the visits were made by female patients. The majority of the visits (87.9%) were made by patients of white race, and most had private insurance (Private=47.6%; Medicaire=34.6%; Medicaid= 4.1%; Selfpay= 4.7%; Other=9.1%) Patient visits from physician's offices that were located in metropolitan statistical areas (MSA) were 82.7%.

From the MEPS dataset (1997 to 2002), 703 million men and women, who were 40 years and older were included. (Table 1) The mean age of these patients was 57.1 years (SD=12.9). About half of the patients (53.2%) were female, and the majority of the patients were of white race (85.4%), had private insurance (75.0%), and were from a MSA (79.4%).(Table 1)

The overall prevalence of vitamin D use during the six year period from NAMCS and MEPS was 0.50% (0.42-0.53) and 0.30% (0.21-0.31), respectively.(Data not shown) In Table 2 the trends in vitamin D use from 1997-2002 are described and each annual prevalence value is reported as the number of subjects or patient visits per 1,000 records. In NAMCS, vitamin D prescriptions were observed in approximately 4-6 of every 1,000 patient visits from 1997-2002.(Table 2) In MEPS the vitamin D use during the six year period was lower than the use noted from NAMCS, as about 2-4 patients per 1,000 subjects had vitamin D prescriptions (Table 2) However, in MEPS it was noted that the prevalence of vitamin D usage increased in 2002 as compared to 1997, while that shown by NAMCS data remained relatively similar over the 6 year period.

Table 1. Characteristics of study population from NAMCS and MEPS 1997 to 2002

Characteristics		NAMCS	MEPS
		N^a (%)[b]	N^a (%)[b]
Total		2,873.6 (100.0)	703.3 (100.0)
Age (years)	40-49	702.6 (24.5)	252.7 (35.9)
	50-59	660.1 (23.0)	185.5 (26.4)
	60-69	578.2 (20.1)	121.0 (17.2)
	70 and over	932.7 (32.5)	144.1 (20.5)
Gender	Female	1,715.7 (59.7)	374.0 (53.2)
	Male	1,157.9 (40.3)	329.4 (46.8)
Race	White	2,526.0 (87.9)	600.6 (85.4)
	Black	248.3 (8.6)	73.1 (10.4)
	Other	99.2 (3.5)	29.6 (4.2)
Insurance	Private	1,369.0 (47.6)	527.6 (75.0)
	Public	1110.6 (38.7)	116.4 (16.5)
	Other[c]	373.9 (13.8)	59.4 (8.4)
Region	Northeast	640.5 (22.3)	139.9 (19.9)
	Midwest	625.5 (21.8)	163.2 (23.2)
	South	945.5 (33.2)	250.3 (35.6)
	West	653.0 (22.7)	150.0 (21.3)
Metropolitan Area	Urban	2,377.4 (82.7)	558.6 (79.4)
	Non-urban	496.2 (17.3)	144.8 (20.6)
Physician specialty[e]	GP/FP	699.2 (24.3)	na[d]
	IM	640.8 (22.3)	na[d]
	OBGY	134.9 (4.7)	na[d]
	All Other	1,398.0 (48.7)	na[d]

[a]Estimates in millions visits for NAMCS and subjects for MEPS
[b]Percentages are based on weighted estimates.
[c]Others represent self-pay or other insurance type from NAMCS and uninsured from MEPS
[d]Not available
[e]GP/FP=general/family practice; IM=internal medicine; OBGY=Obstetrics and Gynecology

**Table 2. Estimated number of records and prevalence
of vitamin D use from 1997 to 2002**

	NAMCS		MEPS	
	N^a	Prevalence[b] (95% CI)	N^a	Prevalence[b] (95% CI)
Vitamin D				
1997	2.0	4.6 (2.8-6.4)	0.2	2.0 (1.2-2.3)
1998	1.7	3.7 (1.9-5.4)	0.3	2.9 (1.8-4.0)
1999	1.6	3.5 (2.6-4.5)	0.2	1.7 (0.7-2.6)
2000	2.7	5.7 (4.1-7.4)	0.3	2.6 (1.3-3.8)
2001	2.8	5.2 (3.4-7.0)	0.3	2.5 (1.6-3.7)
2002	2.9	5.6 (3.8-7.4)	0.5	4.0 (2.6-5.0)

[a]Estimates in millions visits for NAMCS and subjects for MEPS
[b]One in 1000 records

Table 3. Characteristics of vitamin D users from NAMCS 1997 to 2002. (N=90,781)[a]

Visit characteristics	Total	Vitamin D therapy	Prevalence (1 per 1000 visits)
Age			
40-49	21,490	54	2.5
50-59	20,722	47	2.3
60-69	18,362	65	3.5
>=70	30,207	120	4.0
Gender			
Female	51,464	234	4.5
Male	39,317	52	1.3
Race			
White	80,720	255	3.2
Black	7,188	22	3.1
Other	2,873	9	3.1
Pay type			
Private	41,488	119	2.9
Medicare	32,406	132	4.1
Medicaid	3,755	13	3.5
Self-pay	4,835	8	1.7
Other	8,297	14	1.7
Region			
Northeast	19,301	57	3.0
Midwest	19,627	69	3.5
South	30,007	92	3.1
West	21,835	68	3.1
MSA			
MSA	75,595	229	3.0
Non-MSA	15,186	57	2.9
Physician's specialty[b]			
GP/FP	13,681	52	3.8
IM	10,124	69	6.8
OBGY	3,356	41	12.2
All Other	63,620	124	1.9
Osteoporosis diagnosis			
Yes	460	26	56.5
No	90,326	260	2.9

[a]All numbers in the table are based on un-weighted values.
[b]GP/FP=general/family practice; IM=internal medicine; OBGY=Obstetricsand Gynecology

Characteristics of vitamin D users were summarized in Table 3 and Table 4. As some of the estimates were too small to calculate national level estimates with reliability, un-weighted values are used and described in these tables. Of the vitamin D users identified from both databases, there were a higher proportion of female users compared to males (NAMCS 81.8% vs.18.2%; MEPS: 79.5 % vs. 20.5%). In other words, the gender specific prevalence of vitamin D use was significantly higher in females compared to males (NAMCS: 4.5 vs. 1.3 per 1000 visits; MEPS: 4.4 vs. 1.4 per 1000 patients). (Table 3 and Table 4) Based upon age, a higher proportion of vitamin D users were older than 70 (NAMCS: 42.0%; MEPS: 39.1%), and there was a general increased prevalence of use per age category; this trend was observed in NAMCS and MEPS. Also from Tables 3 and 4 the prevalence of vitamin D use among those diagnosed with osteoporosis was higher (NAMCS= 56.5/1000 visits; MEPS =27.3/1000 subjects) compared to those without the condition (NAMCS=2.9/1000 visits; MEPS=2.2/1000 subjects). The overall prevalence of osteoporosis for the entire six year period from NAMCS and MEPS was 0.90% (95% CI 0.75-0.97) and 3.38% (95% CI 3.16-3.61), respectively. (Data not shown) In terms of physician specialty, physicians who specialized in obstetrics and gynecology prescribed the highest rate of vitamin D therapy followed by internal medicine.(Table 3) Vitamin D therapy rates did not differ by the patient's race, MSA status, and geographical region.

Table 4. Characteristics of vitamin D users from MEPS 1997 to 2002. (N=71,356)

Patient characteristics	Total	Vitamin D therapy	Prevalence (1 per 1000 subjects)
Age			
40-49	25,591	36	1.4
50-59	19,116	51	2.7
60-69	12,281	44	3.6
>=70	14,368	84	5.8
Gender			
Female	38,951	171	4.4
Male	32,405	44	1.4
Race			
White	58,694	175	3.0
Black	9,678	28	2.9
Other	2,984	12	4.0
Pay type			
Private	49,596	115	2.3
Public	13,810	82	5.9
Other	7,950	18	2.3
Region			
Northeast	12,761	44	3.4
Midwest	15,300	37	2.4
South	26,919	83	3.1
West	16,376	51	3.1
MSA			
MSA	54,618	41	2.5
Non-MSA	16,738	174	3.2
Osteoporosis diagnosis			
Yes	2,385	65	27.3
No	68,971	150	2.2

[a]All numbers in the table are based on un-weighted values

Based on logistic regression analyses using unweighted values, certain visit characteristics predicted physician's prescription with vitamin D therapy as described in Table 5 and Table 6. Table 5 describes the association between patient visit characteristics and vitamin D therapy using NAMCS. Visits made by patients aged 70 and older were more likely to include a prescription for vitamin D therapy compared to visits made by patients between 40-49 years of age, when unadjusted for other factors.(Table 5).

Table 5. Predictors of vitamin D prescription, NAMCS 1997 to 2002[a]

Visit Characteristics	Unadjusted OR (95% CI)	Adjusted OR (95% CI)
Age		
40-49	Reference (1.00)	Reference (1.00)
50-59	0.90 (0.61,1.34)	0.98 (0.66, 1.45)
60-69	1.41 (0.98, 2.02)	1.49 (1.01, 2.20) [c]
>=70	1.58 (1.14, 2.18) [c]	1.46 (0.96, 2.21)
Gender		
Male	Reference (1.00)	Reference (1.00)
Female	3.45(2.55, 4.66) [c]	2.42 (1.76, 3.34) [c]
Race		
White	Reference (1.00)	Reference (1.00)
Black	0.97 (0.63, 1.50)	0.92 (0.59, 1.43)
Others	0.99 (0.51, 1.93)	0.96 (0.49, 1.91)
Pay type		
Private	Reference (1.00)	Reference (1.00)
Medicare	1.42 (1.11, 1.82) [c]	1.21 (0.86, 1.69)
Medicaid	1.21 (0.68, 2.14)	1.13 (0.63, 2.03)
Self-pay	0.58 (0.28, 1.18)	0.69 (0.34, 1.42)
Other	0.59 (0.34, 1.02)	0.68 (0.39, 1.18)
Region		
Northeast	Reference (1.00)	Reference (1.00)
Midwest	1.19 (0.84, 1.69)	1.20 (0.83, 1.50)
South	1.04 (0.75, 1.45)	1.04 (0.74, 1.45)
West	1.05 (0.74, 1.50)	1.12 (0.78, 1.60)
Metropolitan area		
Urban	Reference (1.00)	Reference (1.00)
Non-urban	0.96 (0.66, 1.41)	1.12(0.83, 1.51)
Physician's specialty[b]		
GP/FP	Reference (1.00)	Reference (1.00)
IM	1.80 (1.25, 2.58) [c]	1.66(1.15, 2.40) [c]
OBGY	3.24 (2.15, 4.89) [c]	2.95(1.92, 4.54) [c]
All Other	0.51 (0.37, 0.71) [c]	0.57(0.41, 0.79) [c]
Osteoporosis diagnosis		
No	Reference (1.00)	Reference (1.00)
Yes	20.76 (13.72, 31.41) [c]	10.53 (6.83, 16.23)[c]

[a]Both un-adjusted and adjusted ORs of likelihood of vitamin D use are based on unweighted values.
[b]GP/FP=general/family practice; IM=internal medicine; OBGY=Obstetrics and Gynecology
[c] $p<0.05$

Patient gender was a predictor for vitamin D use; visits made by female patients were two times more likely to include vitamin D therapy. (Adjusted OR=2.42; 95% CI 1.76-3.34) Physician's specialty was also a strong predictor of vitamin D use. Physicians in internal medicine and practitioners in obstetrics and gynecology were about two and three times more likely to prescribe vitamin D than generalists or other specialists, respectively. (Internal Medicine OR.=1.66; 95% CI 1.15-2.40; Obstetrics and gynecology OR=2.95; 95% CI 1.92-4.54)

We found that the association between vitamin D use and gender was confounded by physician specialty variable. Therefore, subgroup analyses were conducted to assess if the effect of gender were different in each stratum of physician specialty. Our subgroup analyses showed that the crude OR for female was 2.42 (95% CI 1.76-3.34) while stratum-specific OR estimates were 4.62 (95% CI 1.96-10.89) and 4.70 (95% CI 2.33-9.47) within general/family practioners and physicians in internal medicine, respectively. The visits with vitamin D prescription from the obstetrics and gynecology specialists were exclusively made by women. Therefore, in all physician specialty strata, vitamin D prescribing rates were higher in females.

Osteoporosis diagnosis was a strong predictor for vitamin D therapy; as visits made by osteoporosis patients were ten times more likely to be associated with vitamin D therapy than visits without osteoporosis records. (Adjusted OR=10.53; 95% CI 6.83-16.23) However, race, insurance type, geographical region, and MSA status were not significant predictors of vitamin D therapy.

Table 6. Predictors of vitamin D prescription, MEPS 1997 to 2002 [a]

Patient Characteristics	Unadjusted OR (95% CI)	Adjusted OR (95% CI)

Age
  40-49
  50-59
  60-69
  >=70
	Reference (1.00)
	1.90 (1.23, 2.91) [b]
	2.55 (1.64, 3.97) [b]
	4.17 (2.82, 6.17) [b]
		Reference (1.00)
		1.64 (1.07, 2.53) [b]
		1.71 (1.08, 2.71) [b]
		2.13 (1.38, 3.29) [b]

Gender
  Male
  Female
	Reference (1.00)
	3.24 (2.33, 4.51)
		Reference (1.00)
		2.20 (1.56, 3.10) [b]

Race
  White
  Black
  Others
	Reference (1.00)
	1.00 (0.63, 1.61)
	0.96 (0.72, 1.28)
		Reference (1.00)
		1.08 (0.71,1.64)
		1.49 (0.82,2.72)

Pay type
  Private
  Public
  Other
	Reference (1.00)
	2.57 (1.94, 3.41) [b]
	0.98 (0.59, 1.60)
		Reference (1.00)
		1.74 (1.27, 2.37) [b]
		1.30 (0.78, 2.16)

Region
  Northeast
  Midwest
  South
  West
	Reference (1.00)
	0.70 (0.45, 1.10)
	0.89 (0.62, 1.29)
	0.90 (0.60, 1.35)
		Reference (1.00)
		0.83 (0.53,1.29)
		1.01 (0.69,1.46)
		0.99 (0.66,1.49)

Metropolitan area
  Urban
  Non-urban
	Reference (1.00)
	0.77 (0.55, 1.09)
		Reference (1.00)
		0.78 (0.55,1.10)

Osteoporosis diagnosis
  No
  Yes
	Reference (1.00)
	12.85(9.58, 17.25) [b]
		Reference (1.00)
		8.05(5.84, 11.10) [b]

[a]Both un-adjusted and adjusted OR of likelihood of vitamin D use are based on unweighted values.
[b]p<0.05

Multivariate analysis from MEPS yielded similar findings as compared to those from NAMCS. (Table 6) Age was a strong predictor of vitamin D use. Patients who were 60 years and over were about two times more likely to have had a prescription for vitamin D therapy compared to patients who were 40-49 years old. (Adjusted OR=1.71; 95% CI 1.08-2.71 in age 60-69 years old; Adjusted OR=2.13; 95% CI 1.38-3.29 in age 70 and above) (Table 6) Gender and presence of osteoporosis diagnosis also predicted vitamin D use. Female patients were two times more likely than male patients to have a prescription for vitamin D (Adjusted OR=2.20; 95% CI 1.56-3.10); patients with osteoporosis diagnosis were eight times more likely (Adjusted OR=8.05; 95% CI 5.84-11.10) to be associated with vitamin D therapy. (Table 6) Also, vitamin D therapy was associated with insurance type in MEPS, as patients with public insurance were about twice as likely than patients with private insurance to have a vitamin D prescription (Adjusted OR=1.74; 95% CI 1.27-2.37). (Table 6) However, no association was found by patient's race, geographical region, or MSA status.

Discussion

Osteoporotic fractures or kyphosis were previously perceived as unavoidable consequences of aging; however, research has now provided a better understanding of its causes, diagnosis, and more importantly, treatment options. Recently, consensus on the management of osteoporosis has developed emphasizing the identification of individuals at risk with improved prevention, diagnosis, and treatment of osteoporosis with anti-resorptive medications supplemented with calcium/vitamin D for optimal therapy.[5, 7, 9, 28, 29]

A review of the literature highlights several randomized controlled trials demonstrating the efficacy of calcium and vitamin D supplementation on BMD, and reduced fracture risk from falls.[11-15] There is evidence of vitamin D's efficacy on bone density and fractures from clinical trials.[15-18] Earlier findings from Chapuy and colleagues conclude that in a population of 3,270 healthy ambulatory women there was a significant reduction in the number of hip fractures and non-vertebral fractures respectively (43% (p=0.043) and 32% (p=0.015)) in the treatment group, as compared to the placebo group.[13] Also previous study by Dawson and colleagues reported more non-vertebral fractures in the placebo group compared with the treatment group receiving 500mg calcium and 700IU of vitamin D_3 (p=0.02).[12] More recently, results from a UK study involving individuals recruited post hip fracture surgery demonstrated a modest but albeit statistically significant difference in BMD between control and active groups receiving injected vitamin D_3, with and without calcium.[15] Another study by Di Daniele and colleagues reported significant differences between the treatment versus placebo groups after 15 and 30month durations of calcium and vitamin D treatment; the treatment group showed increase in BMD while the placebo group indicated a decrease in BMD(P<0.005) at both intervals.[14]

Though few studies have provided national estimates of vitamin D medication use, there is increasing evidence that vitamin D inadequacies are prevalent among older community dwelling adults.[30-33] Our study, an observational cross sectional study, assessed the vitamin D use in a U.S. ambulatory care setting using national survey data. An epidemiologic study such as this one may provide valuable information regarding how frequently vitamin D is used, and what type of patients are prescribed vitamin D among the U.S. elderly population. In addition, this type of observational studies is an important tool in tracking national trends.

Currently there is limited vitamin D fortification in the US [30] and geriatric adults are at high risk for vitamin D deficiency.[34] Consequently, sun exposure and supplementation remain the only viable nutritional sources.[30] Moreover calcium and vitamin D intake plays a significant role during the post-menopausal period due to the hormonal impact of bone loss.[35] Although our findings indicated an increased trend of vitamin D use from 1997-2002, we believe that the proportion of vitamin D users was still of concern since the study population comprised older adults, potential menopausal women at risk for bone loss, and growing elderly population in the future.

The findings from unweighted analyses showed that there was a higher proportion and higher prevalence of vitamin D use by females and older individuals from both NAMCS and MEPS. These results corroborate the findings of Calvo and colleagues who reported more supplementation with vitamin D by women, and increased use with age in the U.S.[21] Gender is an important risk factor for osteoporotic fracture.[7, 8] As part of a preventative campaign, calcium and vitamin D supplementation is especially encouraged in females.[35] However, a third of all fractures in the older population occur in men [36, 37] and clinical predictors pertaining to falls and frailty are similar for both men and women [38, 39] The current study reports that the prevalence of vitamin D supplementation in men is about 4 times lower than that of women. Moreover regression analysis reports that women were up to 3 times more likely to receive a vitamin D prescription. Based upon previous literature suggesting similar osteoporotic fracture risk in older men, yet underestimation of the disease in men [40, 41], additional use of vitamin D supplementation for fracture prevention in men should be encouraged. In addition, a comprehensive and programmatic approach should be considered targeting both men and women. Other gender related findings from our study pertain to the significance of physician's specialty in the regression model. It was observed that physicians specialized in obstetrics and gynecology were about 3 times more likely to prescribe vitamin D as compared to other generalists and specialists; however as evaluated from the subgroup analysis, physician specialty was identified as a confounding variable affecting gender's effect on vitamin D use. The stratified analysis by physician's specialty also revealed interesting prescribing patterns of vitamin D, as most physicians had increased rates of vitamin D prescribing among females. This observation that physician's in internal medicine, as well as general/family practitioners show such prescribing trends further reveals the need to encourage vitamin D use in men for osteoporosis prevention.

Age is also another important risk factor for osteoporotic fracture.[7, 8] The daily FDA recommendation of vitamin D intake for individuals 51-70yr, and 70 and older are 400IU and 600IU.[30] Our results indicate that the increase in the proportion of vitamin D use is encouraging, as it reflects improving adherence to established practice guidelines. However, in view of the marginal prevalence of vitamin D supplementation, its use should be encouraged among older adults, especially focusing on individuals with higher risk of osteoporotic fracture.

Osteoporosis diagnosis was highly associated with vitamin D use in our study population, in both NAMCS and MEPS. Osteoporosis status was the strongest predictor of vitamin D use, as patients diagnosed were between 8-10 times more likely to be associated with vitamin D supplementation.. With improving focus on concurrent and continued calcium and vitamin D supplementation within optimal osteoporosis management programs, this finding indicates increasing compliance with accepted national treatment guidelines. Additionally this result is significant as it demonstrates that a greater proportion of patients were prescribed the appropriate vitamin D supplementation, after a formal diagnosis compared to patients without the diagnosis.

In interpreting the reported prevalence values, it is important to recognize the differences observed between NAMCS and MEPS estimates for both osteoporosis diagnosis (NAMCS: 0.90% vs. MEPS: 3.38%) and vitamin D use (NAMCS: 0.5% vs. MEPS: 0.3%). This discrepancy could be explained by several factors related to the study design. First, NAMCS and MEPS have different units of observation: the NAMCS's primary sampling unit is a physician office visit while for MEPS it is a patient reported response. Secondly, NAMCS incorporates a multi-stage probability design where the principal sampling units (physician office visits) are documented randomly during an assigned 2 week period.[26, 27] In contrast, the MEPS survey utilizes an overlapping panel design, consisting of six rounds of interviewing over a 2.5 year period.[42] Hence, in the case of NAMCS, it is conceivable that a patient could have multiple visits, if they complete multiple office visits within the two week observation period. Overall, the variations in sampling schemes and observation units in MEPS and NAMCS surveys lead to very distinct study populations. Consequently direct comparison of prevalence estimates between the two surveys may be inappropriate, and variations are best considered from an overall rather than comparative perspective.

Using NAMCS and MEPS data introduces other database specific limitations. First the possibility of truncation in drug records during visits that result in multiple prescriptions cannot be ignored, particularly from NAMCS drug data which may contain only up to six medications. Based on our assessment on the extent of possible truncation bias in NAMCS, about 93.3% of visits received 0 to 5 prescribed medications. Therefore, about 7% of visits were associated with a possibility of bias due to truncated drug records. In MEPS, the prescribed medicine file contains each drug record based on reported prescribed medicine that was purchased or obtained.[43] Unlike NAMCS, MEPS prescribed medicine file allows multiple medication records per patient so that the potential for truncation bias would be extremely low. There is another limitation in the use of MEPS in regard to prescription status of medications. Of the vitamin D compounds, some strengths of ergocalciferol are available without a physician's prescription.[44] Therefore, most of the vitamin D compounds that requires a doctor's prescription would be captured in MEPS. However, the utilization frequencies of vitamin D products that were purchased over-the-counter (OTC) would be potentially underestimated in MEPS. On the other hand, NAMCS contains up to 6 medications that were ordered, supplied, administered or continued during a visit, including prescription and OTC medications.[26, 27] The last consideration relates to clinical and other social factors. These parameters, such as personal preferences or drug coverage status of the patient, cannot be controlled, and could also affect patterns of vitamin D use or osteoporosis diagnosis. In spite of these limitations, our findings may provide a broader representation of vitamin D use, as depicted both by prescribing behavior of physician's from NAMCS and from the patient's perspective using MEPS.

We believe that a coordinated effort through a comprehensive programmatic approach, and continuous communication among health care professionals including; physicians, dentists, nurses, pharmacists, and nutritionists is necessary to improve osteoporosis prevention and treatment. During physician's office visits, primary care physicians can focus on patient counseling regarding calcium and vitamin D supplementation. Although less attention has been focused on the role of dentists regarding osteoporosis management, dentists can be an important resource for identifying initial signs of osteoporosis, and recommend calcium and vitamin D supplementation to prevent further bone loss during visits to dental offices. Potential roles of dentists in screening osteoporosis have been described in previous literature. [45-47] It has also been established that calcium and vitamin D supplementation may slow the rate of bone loss from various skeletal sites. Krall and colleagues [48] reported that subjects taking calcium and vitamin D for osteoporosis prevention exhibited less tooth loss compared to those taking placebo. White and colleagues evaluated the association between clinical and radiographic information during dental office visits and femur BMD.[47] According to their findings, 83% of the individuals with femoral osteopenia or osteoporosis were identified using both clinical and radiographic features.[47] As significant members of the health care team, pharmacists are uniquely positioned and qualified in the healthcare system to provide counseling services on medication adherence and appropriate use of antiresorptive therapies.[49, 50]

In summary, vitamin D plays a significant role in the prevention and treatment of osteoporosis and fragility fracture. In our study population of patients 40 years and older, very few patients were prescribed vitamin D or reported patient visits were associated with vitamin D prescriptions. The overall utilization of vitamin D therapy in the U.S. between1997 and 2002 was suboptimal. As expected, older and female patients, and patients with an osteoporosis diagnosis were more likely to be receiving vitamin D therapy. Our findings support the need for greater awareness on vitamin D supplementation and a coordinated team approach among health care professionals to improve osteoporosis prevention and treatment among individuals who are 40 years and older, especially among men.

Acknowledgements

This study was supported by The Pharmaceutical Research and Manufacturers of American Research Starter Grant Award and grant number 1 R24 HS11673 from the Agency for Healthcare Research and Quality. The authors thank Eric Xue, M.S., biostatistician for the Center for Minority Health Services Research for statistical analyses.

References

[1]   National Osteoporosis Foundation. *Osteoporosis: Fast Facts*. Retrieved July 29, 2005, from *http://www.nof.org/osteoporosis/diseasefacts.htm*

[2]   National Osteoporosis Foundation. Osteoporosis : review of the evidence for prevention, diagnosis, and treatment and cost effective analysis. *Osteoporosis Int* 1998;8:S1-S88

[3]   Cummings SR, Melton LJ. Epidemiology and outcomes of osteoporotic fractures. *Lancet.* 2002;359:1761–7.

[4]   Kessel B. Hip fracture prevention in postmenopausal women. *Obstetrical and Gynecological Survey.* 2004;59(6):446-55

[5]   Physician's guide to prevention and treatment of osteoporosis. Washington D.C.: *National Osteoporosis* Foundation; 2003.

[6]   National Osteoporosis Foundation. *Osteoporosis: Bone basics*. Retrieved July 29, 2005, from *http://www.nof.org/osteoporosis/bonehealth.htm*

[7]   Osteoporosis prevention, diagnosis, and therapy. NIH Consensus Statement. *JAMA* 2001;285:785-95.

[8]   AACE Osteoporosis Task Force. American Association of Clinical Endocrinologists medical guidelines for clinical practice for the prevention and treatment of postmenopausal osteoporosis: 2001 edition, with selected updates for 2003. *Endocrine Practice* 2003;9:544-64

[9]   Consensus development conference: diagnosis, prophylaxis, and treatment of osteoporosis. *Am J Med* 1993;94:646-50.

[10]   Bringhurst FR, Demay MB, Kronenberg HM. Hormones and Disorders of Mineral Metabolism. In: *Larsen PR, et al 10th eds. Williams Textbook of Endocrinology*. St. Louis: W.B. Saunders Co.; 2003:1303-1426.

[11]   Dawson-Hughes B, Harris SS, Krall EA, Dallal GE et al. Rate of bone loss in postmenopausal women randomly assigned to one of two dosages of vitamin D. *American Journal of Clinical Nutrition*. 1995; 61(5):1140-5

[12]   Dawson-Hughes B, Harris SS, Krall EA, Dallal GE et al. Effect of Calcium and Vitamin D Supplementation on Bone Density in Men and women 65 Years of Age or Older. *New England Journal of Medicine*. 1997;337(10):670-676

[13]   Chapuy MC, Arlot ME, Duboeuf F et al. Vitamin D3 and calcium to prevent hip fractures in the elderly. *New England Journal of Medicine*.1992;327(23):1637-42

[14]   Di Daniele N, Carbonelli MG, Candeloro N. Effect if supplementation of calcium and Vitamin D on bone mineral density and bone mineral content in peri-and post – menopause women A double blind, randomized, controlled trial. *Pharmacological Research* 2004;50:637-641

[15]   Harwood RH,Opinder S,Gaynor Ket al. A randomized controlled trial of different calcium and vitamin D supplementation regimens in elderly women after hip fracture The Nottingham Neck of Femur Study: NoNOF Study. *Age and Ageing* 2004;33:45-51

[16]   Ooms ME. Roos JC. Bezemer PD. van der Vijgh WJ. Bouter LM. Lips P. Prevention of bone loss by vitamin D supplementation in elderly women: a randomized double-blind trial. *Journal of Clinical Endocrinology and Metabolism*. 1995;80(4):1052-8

[17]   Heikinheimo RJ, Inkovaara JA, Harju EJ, et al. Annual Injections of Vitamin D and fracture of aged bones. *Calcif Tissue Int*.1992; 51:105-110

[18]   Trivedi DP, Doll R, Khaw KT. Effect of four monthly oral vitamin D3 (cholecalciferol) supplementation on fractures and mortality in men and women living in the community: randomised double blind controlled trial. *BMJ*. 2003;326(7387):469.

[19]   Feskanich D, Willet WC, Graham AC. Calcium, Vitamin D, milk consumption , and hip fractures:a prospective study among postmenopausal women. *Am J Clin Nutr*.2003;77:504-11

[20]   Ness J. Aronow WS. Newkirk E. McDanel D. Underutilization of calcium and vitamin D by older adults in a large general internal medicine practice. *American Journal of Therapeutics*. 2005 12(2):113-6

[21]   Calvo MS. Whiting SJ. Barton CN. Vitamin D intake: a global perspective of current status. *Journal of Nutrition*. 2005 135(2):310-6.

[22]   Lobo RA. Menopause. In: Goldman L, Bennett JC, eds. *Cecil Textbook of Medicine*. Philadelphia: W.B. Saunders Co.; 2000:1360-6.

[23]   Woodwell DA. National Ambulatory Medical Care Survey: 1997 Summary. Hyattsville, MD: National Center for Health Statistics; 1999. *Advance Data from Vital and Health Statistics*. No. 305.

[24]   Cohen SB. Sample design of the 1997 Medical Expenditure Panel Survey Household Component, Rockville (MD): Agency for Healthcare Research and Quality; 2000. *MEPS Methodology* Report No. 11. AHRQ Pub. No. 01-0001.

[25]   Woodwell DA. National Ambulatory Medical Care Survey: 1998 Summary. Hyattsville, MD: National Center for Health Statistics; 2000. *Advance Data from Vital and Health Statistics*. No. 315.

[26]   National Center for Health Statistics. *Public use micro-data file documentation, National Ambulatory Medical Care Survey*, 1997: data and documentation produced by the National Center for Health Statistics. Hyattsville, MD1997.

[27]   National Center for Health Statistics. *Public use micro-data file documentation, National Ambulatory Medical Care Survey*, 1998: data and documentation produced by the National Center for Health Statistics. Hyattsville, MD1998.

[28]   Meunier PJ, Delmas PD, Eastell R et al. Diagnosis and management of osteoporosis in postmenopausal women: clinical guidelines. International Committee for Osteoporosis Clinical Guidelines. *Clin Ther* 1999;21:1025-44.

[29]   Lee E, Zuckerman IH, Weiss SR. Patterns of pharmacotherapy and counseling for osteoporosis management in visits to US ambulatory care physicians by women. *Arch Intern Med*. 2002;162:2362-6.

[30]   Holick MF. Siris ES. Binkley N. Beard MK. Khan A. Katzer JT. Petruschke RA. Chen E. de Papp AE. Prevalence of Vitamin D inadequacy among postmenopausal North American women receiving osteoporosis therapy. *Journal of Clinical Endocrinology and Metabolism*. 2005;90(6):3215-24.

[31]   Levis S. Gomez A. Jimenez C. Veras L. et al. Vitamin D deficiency and seasonal variation in an adult South Florida population. *Journal of Clinical Endocrinology and Metabolism*. 2005 90(3):1557-62.

[32]   Gloth FM, Gundberg CM, Hollis BW, Haddad JG, Tobin JD. Vitamin D deficiency in homebound elderly persons. *JAMA* 1995;274:1683–6.

[33]   Jacques PF, Felson DT, Tucker KL, et al. Plasma 25-hydroxyvitaminD and its determinants in an elderly population sample. *Am J Clin Nutr*. 1997;66:929–36.

[34]   McEvoy GK, Snow EK, Kester L, Miller J, Welsh Jr, OH, Litvak K. editors. *AHFS Drug Information*. Bethesda, MD: American Society of Health-System Pharmacists, Inc. 2005 Chapter 88. Page 3541.

[35]   Wei GS. Jackson JL. Hatzigeorgiou C. Tofferi JK. Osteoporosis management in the new millennium. *Primary Care; Clinics in Office Practice*. 2003;30(4):711-41

[36]   Van Staa TP, Dennison EM, Leufkens HG, Cooper C. Epidemiology of fractures in England and Wales. *Bone*. 2001;29:517–522.

[37]   Jones G, Nguyen TV, Sambrook PN, Kelly PJ, Gilbert C, Eisman JA. Symptomatic fracture incidence in elderly men and women: the Dubbo Osteoporosis Epidemiology Study (DOES). *Osteoporos Int*. 1994;4:277–282.

[38] Center JR, Nguyen TV, Sambrook PN, Eisman JA. Hormonal and biochemical parameters and osteoporotic fractures in elderly men. *J Bone Miner Res.* 2000;15:1405–11.

[39] Tromp AM, Smit JH, Deeg DJ, Bouter LM, Lips P. Predictors for falls and fractures in the Longitudinal Aging Study Amsterdam. *J Bone Miner Res.* 1998;13:1932–9.

[40] Ettinger B. Ray GT. Pressman AR. Gluck O. Limb fractures in elderly men as indicators of subsequent fracture risk. *Archives of Internal Medicine.* 2003;163(22):2741-7.

[41] Meryn S. Undertreatment of osteoporosis in men. *Archives of Internal Medicine.* 2005 165(2):241.

[42] Agency for Health Research and Quality. MEPS HC-031 1999 Full Year Population Characterisitcs. [cited 2005 August 22] Available from *http://meps.ahrq.org/ pubdoc/HC031/H31DOC.htm.*

[43] Agency for Health Research and Quality. MEPS HC-033A 1999 Prescribed Medicine. Dec. 2001. [cited 2005 August 22] Available from *http://www.meps.ahrq.gov/Pubdoc /HC033A/H33Adoc.pdf*

[44] MedlinePlus: Vitamin D and Related Compounds [cited 2005 August 15] Available from *http://www.nlm.nih.gov/medlineplus/druginfo/uspdi/202597.html*

[45] White SC. Oral radiographic predictors of osteoporosis. *Dentomaxillofac Radiol.* 2002; 31(2):84-92

[46] Tozum TF, Tguchi A. role of dental panoramic radiographs in assessment of future dental conditions in patients with osteoporosis and periodontitis. *N Y State Dent J* 2004;70(1):32-5

[47] White SC, Taguchi A, Kao D, Wu S, Service SK, Yoon D, et al. Clinical and panoramic predictors of femur bone mineral density. *Osteoporos Int* 2005;16(3):339-46.

[48] Krall EA, Wehler C, Garcia RI, Harris SS, Dawson-Hughes B. Calcium and vitamin D supplements reduce tooth loss in the elderly. *Am J Med* 2001;111:452-6.

[49] American Pharmacists Association Medication therapy Management Services Working Group. Pharmacy profession stakeholders consensus document; Medication therapy management services definition and program criteria. June 8, 2004.

[50] Medicare prescription drug, improvement, and modernization act of 2003; Public Law 108-173; December 8 2003.

In: Cancer Prevention Research Trends
Editors: Louis Braun and Maximilian Lange

ISBN: 978-1-60456-639-0
© 2008 Nova Science Publishers, Inc.

Chapter IV

Paricalcitol: A Vitamin D2 Analog with Anticancer Effects with Low Calcemic Activity

Takashi Kumagai[1,2] and H. Phillip Koeffler[2]

[1] Department of Hematology, Ohme Municipal General Hospital, Tokyo, Japan
[2] Division of Hematology/Oncology, Department of Medicine Cedars-Sinai Medical Center, Los Angeles, US

Abstract

The use of *all-trans*-retinoic acid (ATRA) for the treatment of acute promyelocytic leukemia shows the power of a non-chemotherapeutic drug to induce the terminal differentiation of leukemia cells. Vitamin D compounds also inhibit the growth of various types of cancers by inducing their differentiation and inhibiting their proliferation *in vitro and vivo*. In a clinical study, orally administrated $1,25(OH)_2D_3$ had modest usefullness for pre-leukemic patients. Because of the calcemic side-effect of $1,25(OH)_2D_3$, the dosage that could be given to these individuals was less than theoretically required for an anticancer effect as noted in vitro. Therefore, new potent, but less calcemic analogs of vitamin D are being synthesized and tested. $19\text{-nor-}1,25(OH)_2D_2$ (Paricalcitol) is a synthetic analogue of $1,25(OH)_2D_2$ currently approved by the FDA for the clinical treatment of secondary hyperparathyroidism in patients with chronic renal failure. This compound has very little calcemic potential as shown by several controlled, randomized clinical trials. Notably, the antiproliferative effects of $19\text{-nor-}1,25(OH)_2D_2$ against human cancers have also recently been reported, including activity against prostate and colon cancers, as well as leukemia and multiple myeloma cells *in vitro* and *in vivo,* associated with cell cycle arrest, induction of differentiation and apoptosis, as well as, decreased expression levels of some tumor suppressor genes. The effect of the analog is mediated through the vitamin D receptor. A clinical trial of paricalcitol has been performed in patients with myelodysplastic syndrome (MDS). Although this therapy was not toxic and hypercalcemia was rarely detected, overall it was not very effective, suggesting that the vitamin vitamin D analog alone may need to be combined with other clinicaly useful drugs.

The combination of vitamin D compounds with other agents have been examined including the addition of the inhibitor of the mitochondrial enzyme, $1,25(OH)_2D_3$ 24-hydroxylase. It is a transcriptional target gene of vitamin D and catalyzes the initial step in the conversion of the active molecule $1,25(OH)_2D_3$ into the less potent metabolite, $1,24,25(OH)_2D_3$. Another example is arsenic trioxide. We have reported that paricalcitol in combination with arsenic trioxide has markedly enhanced anti-myeloid leukemia activity in vitro compared to either agent alone. This may be the case because arsenic trioxide acts as an inhibitor of both 24-hydroxylase as well as the PML-RARα fusion protein, the leukemogenic fusion protein that represses normal blood cell differentiation in this leukemia.

In summary, vitamin D analogs alone may not be potent enough to become a viable anticancer therapy; but when combined with other compounds, they may provide a therapeutic approach to cancers with little toxicity.

Introduction

Cancer chemotherapies are usually toxic for normal cells. On the other hand, induction of differentiation can sometimes be useful as a less toxic therapy that can supplement more aggressive approaches. This approach attempts to remove the cancer cells from the proliferative compartment by inducing it to differentiate into mature, non-dividing cells. This has been most dramatically demonstrated with the use of *all-trans*-retinoic acid (ATRA) for the treatment of acute promyelocytic leukemia. This treatment often induces complete remissions.

1,25-Dihydroxyvitamin D_3 [$1,25(OH)_2D_3$] is a member of the seco-steroid hormone family associated with calcium homeostasis and bone metabolism. $1,25(OH)_2D_3$ can inhibit the growth of various types of cancer cells, including breast, prostate, colon, skin, and brain cancer cells, as well as myeloid leukemia cells. In a clinical study, orally administrated $1,25(OH)_2D_3$ was partially useful for preleukemic patients [1]; but because $1,25(OH)_2D_3$ also causes hypercalcemia, the dose that could be given to these patients was less than that theoretically required for an anticancer effect [2,3]. Consequently, new analogues of vitamin D that are potent, but less calcemic, are being synthesized and tested [4-12].

The 19-nor-1,25-Dihydroxyvitamin D_2 (paricalcitol) is a synthetic analogue of vitamin D that was recently approved by the Food and Drug Administration for the clinical treatment of secondary hyperparathyroidism (Figure 1). It is a white, crystalline powder with the empirical formula of $C27H44O3$, with corresponds to a molecular weight of 417. Paricalcitol is chemically written as 19-nor-1α,3β,25-trihydroxy-9,10-secoergosta-5(Z),7(E),22(E)-triene and has the structural formula as shown in Figure 1. Injectable paricalcitol has been available for use in hemodialysis patients since 1998. It achieves receptor and site selectivity due to modifications to the A ring and the presence of a D_2 side-chain. Rats treated with intravenous paricalcitol demonstrate PTH suppression and less bone resorption than those treated with calcitriol [13,14]. Subsequent studies in hemodialysis patients support the effectiveness of intravenous paricalcitol in controlling secondary hyperparathyroidism in renal failure [13-15]. In a double blind trial, injectable paricalcitol suppressed PTH more rapidly than calcitriol (50% suppression at week 15 versus week 23). Furthermore, paricalcitol caused fewer sustained episodes of hypercalcemia and/or increased calcium-phosphorus product (18% versus 33%; p=0.008). Use of paricalcitol in hemodialysis patients was also associated with a lower hospitalization rate and lower mortality compared to those treated with calcitriol [13]. The survival benefit of paricalcitol was independent of baseline calcium, phosphorus, and PTH levels, and did not correlate with changes in either serum calcium or phosphorus, suggesting other possible beneficial actions. Oral formulation of paricalcitol has increased the convenience of its use and it may also be a less expensive alternative in the hemodialysis population.

Paricalcitol has very little calcemic activity, as demonstrated in randomized controlled clinical trials [16, 17]. Recently, the antiproliferative activity of paricalcitol has been demonstrated in human prostate and colon cancer cells, and human hematological malignancies including acute myeloid leukemia and multiple myeloma cells *in vitro* and *in vivo*. [18-20] (Table 1). So the drug has potential as an anti-cancer agent.

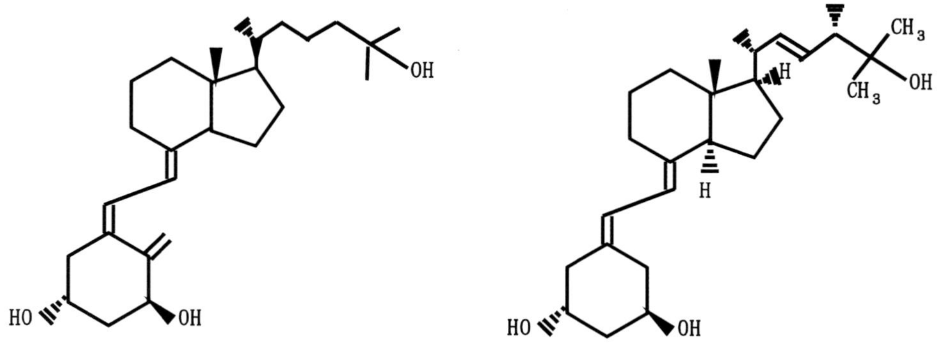

1,25(OH)$_2$D$_3$ 19-Nor-1,25(OH)$_2$D$_2$ (Paricalcitol)

Figure 1. Chemical structures of 1,25(OH)$_2$ Vitamin D$_3$ and paricalcitol (19-Nor-1α, 25(OH)$_2$D$_2$).

Table 1. Preclinical studies of the anti-cancer effects of paricalcitol

Reference	Type of cancer	Combination
Chen et al. (2000)[18]	Prostate (in vitro)	–
Kumagai et al. (2003)[19]	Acute myeloid leukemia (in vitro)	–
	Myeloma (in vitro)	–
	Colon Cancer (in vitro and in vivo)	–
Molnar et al. (2003)[20]	Acute myeloid leukemia (in vitro)	–
Dunlap et al. (2003)[51]	Prostate (in vitro)	Inising radiation
Kumagai et al. (2005)[30]	Acute Myeloid Leukemia (in vitro)	Arsenic trioxide

Anti-Proliferative Activities of Paricalcitol against Human Prostate and Colon Cancers, as well as Myeloid Leukemia and Multiple Myeloma Cells in Vitro and *In Vivo*

The anti-proliferative activity of paricalcitol against prostate cancer cell lines and primary cell cultures was noted initially by Tai C. et al., [18]. It had anti-tumor activity comparable to $1\alpha, 25(OH)_2D_3$ on prostate cancer cell lines and primary cell cultures in vitro. Our group has shown that this compound has anti-cancer activities against myeloid leukemia, myeloma and colon cancer cells in vitro and in vivo, and we explored its mechanism of action against cancer cells [19].

Paricalcitol inhibits the growth of human acute myeloid leukemia (AML) cell lines in vitro at a concentrations in the range of 2-6 x 10^{-9} M resulting in 50% decreased growth (ED50) of HL-60, NB-4 and THP-1 cell lines. Other investigators found similar activity of the compound against HL-60 and U937 AML cells [20]. Exposure of these cells to paricalcitol induced their cell cycle arrest and monocytic differentiation associated with an increased expression of the cyclin dependent kinase inhibitors (CDKIs), $p27^{KIP1}$ and $p21^{WAF1}$, as well as PTEN. Paricalcitol also suppressed the growth of NIH-929 myeloma cells (ED_{50}, 2.0 x 10^{-10} M) with cell cycle arrest, apoptosis, increased expression of $p27^{KIP1}$, and decreased expression of Bcl-2. Paricalcitol suppressed the growth of colon cancer cell lines in vitro (ED_{50}, 1.7 x 10^{-8} M for HT-29 ; 4.6 x 10^{-8} M for SW837) with increased expressions of CDKIs and E-cadherin, and decreased levels of c-myc and cyclin D_1. The analog selectively inhibited COX-2 expression without affecting COX-1 in HT-29 and SW837 in parallel with its anti-proliferative effects. In addition, paricalcitol suppressed the growth of HT-29 colon cancer xenografts growing in mice [19]. The anti-proliferative effect of paricalcitol was comparable to 1,25-dihydroxycholecalciferol [19].

Further studies showed that paricalcitol's effects were probably mediated through the vitamin D receptor (VDR). The analog was able to enhance hematopoietic stem cells from wild type but not VDR-knockout mice to selective differentiation to macrophages, suggesting it mediated its differentiation effects through VDR [19].

Of interest, the peak concentration of paricalcitol in patients with chronic renal failure was 4.4 ± 1.6 x 10^{-9} M after intravenous dose of 0.24 g/kg [21]. This concentration does not result in hypercalcemia in most patients and it is currently the recommended maximum dose in the treatment of secondary hyperparathyroidism. This concentration is adequate for a moderate anti-proliferative effect of paricalcitol against vitamin D-sensitive cancer cells; and higher blood plasma concentrations are achievable with further dose escalation. Taken together, these studies prompted us to do a clinical trial using paricalcitol.

Clinical Trials of Vitamin D and Its Analogs

Even though in vitro studies by our laboratory and others have demonstrated that $1,25(OH)_2D_3$ and its analogs show promise against cancer cells, clinical trials of vitamin D compounds in leukemia and myelodysplastic syndrome (MDS) have so far yielded mediocre results.

One of the first trials of $1,25(OH)_2D_3$ to treat MDS was performed by us [1]. Eighteen individuals with MDS were given $1,25(OH)_2D_3$ at 2 µg/day for approximately 12 weeks. Eight patients had either a partial or minor response whereby their peripheral blood granulocytes, platelets and macrophage counts were slightly elevated compared to their baseline values. However, none showed significant improvement in their cell counts at the end of the study. Seven individuals developed leukemia, and nine out of 18 patients developed hypercalcemia.

Another clinical trial involved six patients with myelodysplastic syndrome (MDS) treated with $1\alpha(OH)$ D3 at 1 µg/day for a minimum of 3 months [22]. The outcome of the trial showed neither a good clinical response nor toxicity in any of the individuals. A third clinical trial [23] consisted of 30 MDS patients, half of these treated with 1α (OH) D3 at 4–6 µg/day for a median of 17 weeks and the remaining patients given a placebo. An improvement in hematopoietic parameters was detected in only one patient receiving the vitamin D compound. However, the investigators felt that the treated group contained a greater proportion of patients that did not progress to leukemia compared to the control group. Hypercalcemia and increased serum creatine levels were observed in two individuals. These parameters regressed when the dose was reduced. We performed a trial of oral paricalcitol for the treatment of MDS. Eleven of the 12 individuals were dependent on red cell transfusions. Each patient was elderly, and most had a poor prognosis. They were given an average dose of 16 µg/day paricalcitol (range 4–56 µg/day) over about 4 months. No toxicity was observed, and one patient had a partial response with his platelet count rising from 50,000 μl^{-1} of blood to the normal range. Although this therapy was not toxic, overall it was not very effective [24].

Lowe et al., gave high dose weekly oral calcitriol (0.5 µg/kg) to patients with prostate cancer who maintained a reduced calcium diet [25]. Three out of 22 patients had confirmed reductions in the serum PSA, a marker of the disease. High dose weekly paricalcitol therapy may be an interesting approach to explore further.

Overall, these clinical trials provide tempered enthusiasm that vitamin D analogs have anti-cancer effect in patients with malignancy, and these analogs have fewer calcemic side-effects. But the data also showed that a vitamin D compound alone may not have sufficient anti-tumor potency.

Paricalcitol in Combination with Other Clinical Useful Drugs

A poor response to a single agent like a vitamin D analog for MDS patients may not be too surprising, because the pathogenesis of this collection of diseases is usually multi-factorial, not being explained by a single molecular target. In contrast, a successful molecular targeted agent like ATRA or imanitib has a clear molecular target such as PML-RAR or BCR-ABL, which are the major pathogenetic abnormalities of APL and CML, respectively.

Pre-clinical studies suggest that the combination of either $1,25(OH)(2)D3$ or its analogs with other agents can have either additive or synergistic anti-cancer activities, suggesting future clinical studies. For example, our group reported that the 20-epi vitamin D analogs and 9-cis retinoic acid had dramatic synergestic anti-proliferative activity against APL cells by inducing granulocytic and monocytic differentiation [26]. Also, one of the novel vitamin D analogs combined with paclitaxel, cisplatin and all-trans-retinoic acid had strong anti-proliferative effects against human breast cancer cells growing in nude mice in vivo [27-29]. We have reported that paricalcitol combined with either arsenic trioxide or dexamethasone have synergistic anti-proliferative effects againt myeloid leukemia and myeloma cells, respectively [30].

During the last decade, the efficiency of AS_2O_3 has been established for both newly diagnosed and relapsed patients with APL. It can be used as a single agent and induces complete remissions with only minimal myelosupression [31]. The NB-4 acute promyelocytic leukemia cell line is a good model for APL having the prerequisite t[15;17] chromosomal translocation specific for APL. In our study, paricalcitol when combined with AS_2O_3, greatly suppressed the growth of NB-4 cells by inducing monocytic differentiation and subsequent apoptosis, while paricalcitol alone was unable to stimulate monocytic differentiation of these cells.

The enhanced activity of paricalcitol presence of arsenic trioxide against acute promyelocytic leukemia cells may be explained by the latter's ability to inhibit the mitochondrial enzyme, 24-hydroxylase and cause the rapid degradation of the PML-RAR fusion protein expressed in acute promyelocytic leukemia cells.

The 25-hydroxyvitamin D_3-24-hydroxylase is the enzyme responsible for the first step in the catabolism of $1,25(OH)_2D_3$ [32]. Transcriptional induction of expression of 24-hydroxylase is dependent on ligand activation of VDR which heterodimerizes with RXR and this activated complex binds to the vitamin D response element of the promoter of the 24-hydroxylase gene [33,34]. This mitchondrial enzyme catalyzes the initial step in the conversion of the active molecule, $1,25(OH)_2D_3$, into the less active metabolite, $1,24,25(OH)_2D_3$ resulting in the inhibition of the anti-proliferative effects of vitamin D [35-38]. In fact, 24-hydroxylase has been suggested to be an oncogene [38]. Thus, an inhibitor of 24-hydroxylase can enhance the effect of vitamin D. The combination of a vitamin D compound and an inhibitor of 24-hydroxylase, such as either genistein, isoflavone or ketoconazole may be a useful approach to cancer therapy [39-42].

Although transcription of 24-hydroxylase was activated by paricalcitol and was rather enhanced by AS_2O_3, the enzyme activity of 24-hydroxylase in mitochondria was decreased by AS_2O_3 in HL-60 and NB-4 cells [30]. This is probably because AS_2O_3 inhibits intracellular 24-hydroxylase activity by disrupting mitochondrial integrity, resulting in higher intracellular levels of the vitamin D analog [30] (Figure 2). Prior studies have shown that the PML-RARα fusion protein impairs differentiation in response to vitamin D *in vitro* and *in vivo* [43-45]. This block of differentiation is thought to occur by the aberrant recruitment of co-repressor proteins and histone deacetylases by PML-RARα, and perhaps by direct sequestering of the vitamin D_3 receptor [45, 46].

Arsenic enhances the degradation of the PML-RARα by promoting the binding of SUMO to the fusion protein [47, 48]. Also, AS_2O_3 rapidly inhibits the interaction of the SMRT corepressor with the PML-RARα fusion protein leading to the reduction of the repression of retinoid target genes [49]. In addition, a recent study suggests that AS_2O_3 increases acetylation of histones H3 and H4 leading to gene activation [50].

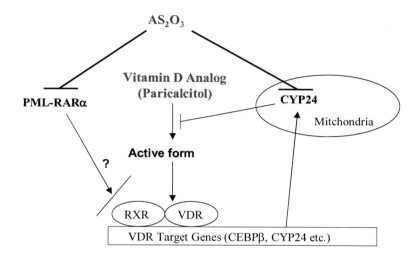

Figure 2. Proposed mechanism of the anti-proliferative effect of paricalcitol and AS_2O_3 against acute myeloid leukemia cells.

Our study showed that the AS_2O_3-enhanced differentiation mediated by paricalcitol was associated with a decreased protein expression of PML-RARα in NB-4 cells and U937-PR9 cells containing a zinc-inducible PML-RARα expression vector, suggesting that the degradation of this fusion protein by AS_2O_3 has an important role for the enhanced response to paricalcitol (Figure 2). Therefore, targeting of the fusion protein might be important in allowing vitamin D compounds to induce differentiation.

A clinical trial of paricalcitol with AS_2O_3 may be a useful approach for APL patients resistant to ATRA.

Conclusion

Vitamin D compounds have been reported to have anti-tumor activities against many cancers in vitro, and its hypercalcemic side-effect has been mitigated by the development of analogs such as paricalcitol. But clinical trials showed that $1,25(OH)_2$ vitamin D_3 or its analogs including paricalcitol alone have limited activity against cancer. Therefore, as is the case for chemotherapeutic drugs, the combination of the vitamin D analog with other clinical useful drugs may enhance anticancer responses. Combinations, such as paricalcitol and AS_2O_3, may provide a therapeutic approach with limited toxicity.

References

[1]   Koeffler HP, Hirji K, Itri L. 1,25-Dihydroxyvitamin D3: in vivo and in vitro effects on human preleukemic and leukemic cells. *Cancer Treat Rep* 1985;69:1399-407.

[2]   Staquet MJ, Byar DP, Green SB, Rozencweig M. Clinical predictivity of transplantable tumor systems in the selection of newdrugs for solid tumors: reply to a commentary. *Cancer Treat Rep* 1985;69:1339-40.

[3]   Koeffler HP, Amatruda T, Ikekawa N, Kobayashi Y, DeLuca HF. Induction of macrophage differentiation of human normal and leukemic myeloid stem cells by 1,25-dihydroxyvitamin D3 and its fluorinated analogues. *Cancer Res* 1984;44:5624-8.

[4]   Abe J, Nakano T, Nishii Y, Matsumoto T, Ogata E, Ikeda K. A novel vitamin D3 analog, 22-oxa-1,25-dihydroxyvitamin D3, inhibits the growth of human breast cancer in vitro and in vivo without causing hypercalcemia. *Endocrinology* 1991;129:832-7.

[5]   Zhou JY, Norman AW, Akashi M, Chen DL, Uskokovic MR, Aurrecoechea JM et al. Development of a novel 1,25(OH)2-vitamin D3 analog with potent ability to induce HL-60 cell differentiation without modulating calcium metabolism. *Blood* 1991;78:75-82.

[6]   Jung SJ, Lee YY, Pakkala S, de Vos S, Elstner E, Norman AW, et al. 1,25(OH)2-16-ene-vitamin D3 is a potent antileukemic agent with low potential to cause hypercalcemia. *Leuk Res* 1994;18:453-63.

[7]   Anzano MA, Smith JM, Uskokovic MR, Peer CW, Mullen LT, Letterio JJ, et al. 1 alpha,25-Dihydroxy-16-ene-23-yne-26,27-hexafluorocholecalciferol (Ro24-5531), a new deltanoid (vitamin D analogue) for prevention of breast cancer in the rat. *Cancer Res* 1994;54:1653-6.

[8]   Pakkala S, de Vos S, Elstner E, Rude RK, Uskokovic M, Binderup L, et al. Vitamin D3 analogs: effect on leukemic clonal growth and differentiation, and on serum calcium levels. *Leuk Res* 1995;19:65-72.

[9]   Koike M, Elstner E, Campbell MJ, Asou H, Uskokovic M, Tsuruoka N, et al. 19-nor-hexafluoride analogue of vitamin D3: a novel class of potent inhibitors of proliferation of human breast cell lines. *Cancer Res* 1997;57:4545-50.

[10]   Kubota T, Koshizuka K, Koike M, Uskokovic M, Miyoshi I, Koeffler HP. 19-nor-26,27-bishomo-vitamin D3 analogs: a unique class of potent inhibitors of proliferation of prostate, breast, and hematopoietic cancer cells. *Cancer Res* 1998;58:3370-5.

[11]   Hisatake J, Kubota T, Hisatake Y, Uskokovic M, Tomoyasu S, Koeffler HP. 5,6-trans-16-ene-vitamin D3: a new class of potent inhibitors of proliferation of prostate, breast, and myeloid leukemic cells. *Cancer Res* 1999;59:4023-9.

[12]   Hisatake J, O'Kelly J, Uskokovic MR, Tomoyasu S, Koeffler HP. Novel vitamin D(3) analog, 21-(3-methyl-3-hydroxy-butyl)-19-nor D(3), that modulates cell growth, differentiation, apoptosis, cell cycle, and induction of PTEN in leukemic cells. *Blood* 2001;97:2427-33.

[13] Holliday LS, et al. 1,25-Dihydroxy-19-nor-vitamin D (2), a vitamin D analog with reduced bone resorbing activity in vitro. *J Am Soc Nephrol* (2000); 11: 1857-1864.

[14] Finch JL, Brown AJ, Slatopolsky E. Differential effects of 1,25-dihydroxy-vitamin D3 and 19-nor-1,25-dihydroxy-vitamin-D2 on calcium and phosphorus resorption in bone. *J Am Soc Nephrol* (1999); 10: 980-985.

[15] Martin KJ. Paricalcitol dosing according to body weight or severity of hyperparathyroidism: a double blind, multicenter, radomized study. Am *J Kidney Dis (2001)*; 38 Supplemental: S57-S63.

[16] Llach F, Keshav G, Goldblat MV, Lindberg JS, Sadler R, Delmez J, et al. Suppression of parathyroid hormone secretion in hemodialysis patients by a novel vitamin D analogue: 19-nor-1,25-dihydroxyvitamin D2. *Am J Kidney Dis* 1998;32(2 Suppl 2):S48-54.

[17] Martin KJ, Gonzalez EA, Gellens M, Hamm LL, Abboud H, Lindberg J. 19-Nor-1-alpha-25-dihydroxyvitamin D2 (Paricalcitol) safely and effectively reduces the levels of intact parathyroid hormone in patients on hemodialysis. *J Am Soc Nephrol* 1998;9:1427-32.

[18] Chen TC, Schwartz GG, Burnstein KL, Lokeshwar BL, Holick MF. The in vitro evaluation of 25-hydroxyvitamin D3 and 19-nor-1alpha,25-dihydroxyvitamin D2 as therapeutic agents for prostate cancer. *Clin Cancer Res* 2000;6:901-8.

[19] Kumagai T, O'Kelly J, Said JW, Koeffler HP. Vitamin D2 analog 19-nor-1,25-dihydroxyvitamin D2: antitumor activity against leukemia, myeloma, and colon cancer cells. *J Natl Cancer Inst*. 2003 Jun 18;95(12):896-905.

[20] Molnar I, Kute T, Willingham MC, Powell BL, Dodge WH, Schwartz GG. 19-nor-1alpha,25-dihydroxyvitamin D(2) (paricalcitol): effects on clonal proliferation, differentiation, and apoptosis in human leukemic cell lines. *J Cancer Res Clin Oncol*. 2003 Jan;129(1):35-42. Epub 2003 Feb 12.

[21] Product information: Zemplar (TM), *paricalcitol, Abbot Laboratories*, North Chicago, IL, 1998

[22] A. Metha, T. Kumaran, G. Marsh, Treatment of myelodysplastic syndrome with alfacacidol, *Lancet* 2 (1984) 761.

[23] S. Motomura, H. Kanamori, A. Maruta, F. Kodama, T. Ohkubo, The effect of 1-hydroxyvitamin D3 for prolongation of leukemic transformation-free survival in myelodysplastic syndromes, *Am. J. Hematol.* 38 (1991) 67–68.

[24] H.P. Koeffler, N. Aslanian, Southern California Leukemia Group, J. O'Kelly, Vitamin D2 analog (Paricalcitol; Zemplar) for treatment of myelodysplastic syndrome, *Leukemia Res.* (2005) in press.

[25] Bruce A Lowe, W D Henner, Dianne D Lemmon, Rakhee Urankar, Tomasz M Beer Long term administration of high dose weekly oral calcitriol in patients with a rising PSA after definitive treatment for prostate cancer (PC): *a phase II study. 2002 ASCO Annual Meeting* Abstract No. 2446

[26] Elstner E, Linker-Israeli M, Le J, Umiel T, Michl P, Said JW, Binderup L, Reed JC, Koeffler HP. Synergistic decrease of clonal proliferation, induction of differentiation, and apoptosis of acute promyelocytic leukemia cells after combined treatment with novel 20-epi vitamin D3 analogs and 9-cis retinoic acid. *J Clin Invest*. 1997 ;99(2):349-60.

[27]   Koshizuka K, Koike M, Asou H, Cho SK, Stephen T, Rude RK, Binderup L, Uskokovic M, Koeffler HP. Combined effect of vitamin D3 analogs and paclitaxel on the growth of MCF-7 breast cancer cells in vivo. *Breast Cancer Res Treat.* 1999 ;53(2):113-20.

[28]   Koshizuka K, Kubota T, Said J, Koike M, Binderup L, Uskokovic M, Koeffler HP. Combination therapy of a vitamin D3 analog and all-trans-retinoic acid: effect on human breast cancer in nude mice. *Anticancer Res.* 1999 ;19(1A):519-24.

[29]   Koshizuka K, Koike M, Kubota T, Said J, Binderup L, Koeffler HP. Novel vitamin D3 analog (CB1093) when combined with paclitaxel and cisplatin inhibit growth of MCF-7 human breast cancer cells in vivo. *Int J Oncol.* 1998 ;13(3):421-8.

[30]   Kumagai T, Shih LY, Hughes SV, Desmond JC, O'Kelly J, Hewison M, Koeffler HP. 19-Nor-1,25(OH)2D2 (a novel, noncalcemic vitamin D analogue), combined with arsenic trioxide, has potent antitumor activity against myeloid leukemia. *Cancer Res.* 2005 ;65(6):2488-97.

[31]   Zhang P., Wang S., and Hu X.H. Arsenic trioxide treated 72 cases of acute promyelocytic leukemia. *Chinese Journal of Hematology.*, 17: 58-62, 1996

[32]   Jones G, Strugnell SA, DeLuca HF. Current understanding of the molecular actions of vitamin D. *Physiol Rev.* 1998;78:1193-231.

[33]   Zierold C, Darwish HM, DeLuca HF. Identification of a vitamin D-response element in the rat calcidiol (25-hydroxyvitamin D3) 24-hydroxylase gene. *Proc Natl Acad Sci U S A.* 1994;91(3):900-2.

[34]   Ohyama Y, Ozono K, Uchida M, et al. Identification of a vitamin D-responsive element in the 5'-flanking region of the rat 25-hydroxyvitamin D3 24-hydroxylase gene. *J Biol Chem.* 1994;269(14):10545-50.

[35]   Krishnan AV, Peehl DM, Feldman D. Inhibition of prostate cancer growth by vitamin D: Regulation of target gene expression. *J Cell Biochem.* 2003 ;88(2):363-71.

[36]   Krishnan AV, Peehl DM, Feldman D. The role of vitamin D in prostate cancer. *Recent Results Cancer Res.* 2003;164:205-21.

[37]   Peehl DM, Krishnan AV, Feldman D. Pathways mediating the growth-inhibitory actions of vitamin D in prostate cancer. *J Nutr.* 2003;133(7 Suppl):2461S-2469S.

[38]   Albertson DG, Ylstra B, Segraves R, et al. Quantitative mapping of amplicon structure by array CGH identifies CYP24 as a candidate oncogene. *Nat Genet.* 2000 ;25(2):144-6.

[39]   Farhan H, Wahala K, Adlercreutz H, Cross HS. Isoflavonoids inhibit catabolism of vitamin D in prostate cancer cells. *J Chromatogr B Analyt Technol Biomed Life Sci.* 2002 ;777:261-8.

[40]   Farhan H, Cross HS. Transcriptional inhibition of CYP24 by genistein. *Ann N Y Acad Sci.* 2002;973:459-62.

[41]   Krishnan AV, Peehl DM, Feldman D. The role of vitamin D in prostate cancer. *Recent Results Cancer Res.* 2003;164:205-21. Review.

[42]   Peehl DM, Seto E, Hsu JY, Feldman D. Preclinical activity of ketoconazole in combination with calcitriol or the vitamin D analogue EB 1089 in prostate cancer cells. *J Urol.* 2002 Oct;168(4 Pt 1):1583-8.

[43]   Ruthardt M, Testa U, et al. Opposite effects of the acute promyelocytic leukemia PML-retinoic acid receptor alpha (RAR alpha) and PLZF-RAR alpha fusion proteins on retinoic acid signalling. *Mol Cell Biol.* 1997;17:4859-69.

[44] Rego EM, Wang ZG, Peruzzi D, He LZ, Cordon-Cardo C, Pandolfi PP. Role of promyelocytic leukemia (PML) protein in tumor suppression. *J Exp Med.* 2001 ;193:521-29.

[45] Puccetti E, Obradovic D, Beissert T, et al. AML-associated translocation products block vitamin D(3)-induced differentiation by sequestering the vitamin D(3) receptor. *Cancer Res.* 2002;62:7050-8.

[46] Grignani F, De Matteis S, Nervi C, et al. Fusion proteins of the retinoic acid receptor-alpha recruit histone deacetylase in promyelocytic leukaemia. *Nature.* 1998;391:815-8.

[47] Zhu J, Lallemand-Breitenbach V, de The H. Pathways of retinoic acid- or arsenic trioxide-induced PML/RARalpha catabolism, role of oncogene degradation in disease remission. *Oncogene.* 2001;20:7257-65.

[48] Seeler JS, Dejean A. SUMO: of branched proteins and nuclear bodies. *Oncogene.* 2001;20:7243-9.

[49] Hong SH, Yang Z, Privalsky ML. Arsenic trioxide is a potent inhibitor of the interaction of SMRT corepressor with Its transcription factor partners, including the PML-retinoic acid receptor alpha oncoprotein found in human acute promyelocytic leukemia. *Mol Cell Biol.* 2001;21:7172-82

[50] Chen Z, Chen GQ, Shen ZX, Chen SJ, Wang ZY. Treatment of acute promyelocytic leukemia with arsenic compounds: in vitro and in vivo studies. *Semin Hematol.* 2001;38:26-36.

[51] Dunlap N, Schwartz GG, Eads D, Cramer SD, Sherk AB, John V, Koumenis C. 1alpha,25-dihydroxyvitamin D(3) (calcitriol) and its analogue, 19-nor-1alpha,25(OH)(2)D(2), potentiate the effects of ionising radiation on human prostate cancer cells. *Br J Cancer.* 2003 Aug 18;89(4):746

In: Cancer Prevention Research Trends
Editors: Louis Braun and Maximilian Lange

ISBN: 978-1-60456-639-0
© 2008 Nova Science Publishers, Inc.

Chapter V

Reduction in the Risk of Human Breast Cancer by Selective Cyclooxygenase-2 (COX-2) Inhibitors: Final Results of a Case Control Study

Randall E. Harris[*]*, Joanne Beebe-Donk and Galal A. Alshafie*
The Ohio State University College of Medicine and Public Health
320 West 10th Avenue
Columbus, Ohio, USA 43210-1240

Abstract

Background

Epidemiologic and laboratory investigations suggest that nonsteroidal anti-inflammatory drugs (NSAIDs) have chemopreventive effects against breast cancer due to their activity against cyclooxygenase-2 (COX-2), the rate-limiting enzyme of the prostaglandin cascade.

Methods

We conducted a case control study of breast cancer designed to compare effects of selective and non-selective COX-2 inhibitors. A total of 611 incident breast cancer patients were ascertained from the James Cancer Hospital, Columbus, Ohio, during 2003-2004 and compared with 615 cancer free controls frequency-matched to the cases on age, race, and county of residence. Data on the past and current use of prescription and over the counter medications and breast cancer risk factors were ascertained using a standardized risk factor questionnaire. Effects of COX-2 inhibiting agents were quantified by calculating odds ratios (OR) and 95% confidence intervals.

Results

Results showed significant risk reductions for selective COX-2 inhibitors as a group (OR=0.15, 95% CI=0.08-0.28), regular aspirin (OR=0.46, 95% CI = 0.32-0.65), and ibuprofen or naproxen (0.36, 95% CI= 0.21-0.60). Intake of COX-2 inhibitors produced significant risk reductions for premenopausal women (OR=0.05), postmenopausal women (OR=0.26), women with a positive family history (OR=0.19), women with a negative family history (OR=0.14), women with estrogen receptor positive tumors (OR=0.24), women with estrogen receptor negative tumors (OR=0.05), women with HER-2/neu positive tumors (OR=0.26), and women with HER-2/neu negative tumors (OR=0.17). Acetaminophen, a compound with negligible COX-2 activity produced no significant change in the risk of breast cancer.

Conclusions

Selective COX-2 inhibitors (celecoxib and rofecoxib) were only recently approved for use in 1999, and rofecoxib (Vioxx) was withdrawn from the marketplace in 2004. Nevertheless, even in the short window of exposure to these compounds, the selective COX-2 inhibitors produced a significant (85%) reduction in the risk of breast cancer, underscoring their strong potential for breast cancer chemoprevention.

Background

The recent recall of rofecoxib (Vioxx) from the marketplace due its alleged association with increased risk for cardiovascular disease has severely compromised further testing of all selective cyclooxygenase-2 (COX-2) inhibitors in the chemoprevention and therapy of cancer. Despite compelling evidence that COX-2 inhibitors have powerful anti-cancer effects, several clinical trials designed to evaluate these compounds in the chemoprevention and therapy of neoplasms have been discontinued or suspended [1, 2].

Both the magnitude and the direction of effect of selective COX-2 blockers on the risk of cardiovascular disease is the subject of controversy. Risk increases have been observed with use of rofecoxib and celecoxib in clinical trials that were designed to evaluate their potential for treating arthritis or reducing colonic polyp recurrence [3, 4, 5], whereas risk decreases have been observed in observational studies that were designed to evaluate effects of these same compounds on cardiovascular diseases [6, 7, 8]. Still other investigations suggest that COX-2 inhibitors have no effect on the risk of myocardial infarction and related cardiovascular events [9, 10].

Among American women, breast cancer is the most frequently diagnosed malignancy and second leading cause of cancer death [11]. Despite intensive efforts aimed primarily at early detection and therapy, the mortality rates of breast cancer have remained virtually constant for several decades. Innovative research efforts must therefore be redirected towards chemoprevention of the early stages of carcinogenesis. Among twenty published epidemiologic studies that focused on the association between intake of nonsteroidal anti-inflammatory drugs (NSAIDs) and the risk of human breast cancer, 13 reported statistically significant risk reductions. Meta-analysis of these data suggests that regular NSAID intake significantly reduces the risk of breast cancer [12].

Two selective COX-2 inhibitors, celecoxib (Celebrex) and rofecoxib (Vioxx), were approved for the treatment of arthritis by the United States Food and Drug Administration (FDA) in 1999. Until the recall of Vioxx in September, 2004, these two compounds plus other selective COX-2 inhibitors valdecoxib (Bextra) and meloxicam (Mobic) were widely utilized in the United States for pain relief and treatment of osteoarthritis and rheumatoid arthritis. The time period between approvals of Celebrex to the recall of Vioxx provides an approximate six-year window for evaluation of exposure to such compounds by a case control approach. The current case control study was designed to test the chemopreventive value of selective COX-2 blockade against human breast cancer.

Methods

We studied 611 cases of invasive breast cancer with histological verification based upon review of the pathology records, and 615 group-matched controls with no personal history of cancer and no current breast disease based on screening mammography. Cases were sequentially ascertained for interview at the time of their diagnosis during 2003 through September, 2004 at The Arthur G. James Cancer Hospital and Richard J. Solove Research Institute (CHRI), Columbus, Ohio. There were no refusals to participate among cases. The controls were ascertained from the mammography service of the cancer hospital during the same time period and frequency matched to the cases by five-year age interval, race, and place (county) of residence. Controls were sequentially ascertained for each matching category resulting in a stratified random sample. Among women eligible for participation, 95% completed the questionnaire.

Critical information on exposure to NSAIDs and other factors were obtained utilizing a standardized risk factor questionnaire. The questionnaires were administered in person by trained medical personnel prior to definitive surgery or treatment for the cases and at the time of screening mammography for controls. The data variables collected consisted of demographic characteristics, height, weight, menstrual and pregnancy history, family history of breast and ovarian cancer, comprehensive information on cigarette smoking, alcohol intake, pre-existing medical conditions (arthritis, chronic headache, cardiovascular conditions including hypertension, angina, ischemic attacks, stroke, and myocardial infarction, lung disease, and diabetes mellitus), and medication history including over the counter (OTC) and prescription NSAIDs, and exogenous hormones. Regarding selective COX-2 inhibitors and other NSAIDs, the use pattern (frequency, dose, and duration), and the type, (celecoxib, valdecoxib, rofecoxib, meloxicam, aspirin, ibuprofen, naproxen, indomethacin) were recorded. Data on the related analgesic, acetaminophen were collected for comparison with selective COX-2 inhibitors and other NSAIDs.

Case-control differences in means and frequencies were checked for statistical significance by t-tests and chi square tests, respectively. Effects of the selective COX-2 inhibitors as a group were quantified by estimating odds ratios and their 95% confidence intervals. Odds ratios were adjusted for age and classical breast cancer risk factors (parity, family history, body mass, menopausal status, chronic smoking, and regular alcohol intake) by logistic regression analysis [13, 14]. Adjusted estimates were obtained for specific types of compounds, e.g., over the counter NSAIDs, selective COX-2 inhibitors, and acetaminophen.

Estimates for selective COX-2 inhibitors were checked for stability by conducting subgroup analyses by menopausal status, family history, and estrogen receptor and human epidermal growth factor receptor (HER-2/neu) status.

Results

Pertinent characteristics of the cases and controls are given in Table 1. The cases exhibited higher frequencies of nulliparity, family history of breast or ovarian cancer, estrogen replacement therapy in postmenopausal subjects, and chronic cigarette smoking. As expected, cases and controls had similar distributions of age, race, and education.

Table 1. Characteristics of breast cancer cases and controls.

Characteristic [a]	Cases (N=323)	Controls (N=649)
Age (yrs)		
<50	19%	20 %
50-65	55	52
>65	26	28
Mean (SEM)	55.8 (0.8)	55.2 (0.4)
Race		
Caucasian	91 %	89 %
All Other	9	11
Education		
< 12 yrs	12 %	12 %
12 yrs	53	55
> 12 yrs	31	33
Parity		
Nulliparous	6 %	4 %
First Pregnancy <30 yrs	83	89
First Pregnancy >30 yrs	11	7 (p<0.05)
Family History		
Positive	32 %	17 %
Negative	68	83 (p<0.01)
Body Mass		
BMI < 22	23 %	21 %
BMI 22-28	35	39
BMI > 28	42	40
Mean (SEM)	27.5 (0.9)	27.1 (0.7)
Menopausal Status		
Premenopausal	41 %	47 %
Postmenopausal	52	53
Postmenopausal ERT	38	31 (p<0.05)
Smoking		
Never smoker	35 %	32 %
Ex-smoker	38	40
Current smoker	27	28
Alcohol Intake		
None	47 %	45 %
1-2 drinks per week	36	35
> 2 drinks per week	17	20

[a] Family History: either breast or ovarian cancer among first or second degree female relatives; ERT=Estrogen Replacement Therapy for two or more years; Body Mass Index = weight (kg) / ht ^{2} (m).

Table 2 shows the comparative frequencies of the medications under study with odds ratios and 95% confidence intervals. Multivariate-adjusted estimates are presented. A significant reduction in the risk of breast cancer was observed for daily intake of selective COX-2 inhibitors for two years or more (OR=0.15, 95% CI=0.08-0.28). Observed risk reductions were consistent for the individual COX-2 inhibitors, celecoxib (OR=0.14, 95% CI=0.05-0.43) and rofecoxib (OR=0.15, 95% CI= 0.06-0.37). Significant risk reductions were also observed for the intake of two or more pills per week of aspirin (OR=0.46, 95% CI= 0.32-0.65) and ibuprofen or naproxen (OR=0.36, 95% CI=0.21-0.60). Acetaminophen, an analgesic with negligible COX-2 activity had no effect on the relative risk of breast cancer (OR=0.98, 95% CI=0.53-1.82).

Table 2. Odds ratios with 95% confidence intervals for breast cancer and selective cyclooxygenase-2 (COX-2) inhibitors, and over the counter nonsteroidal anti-inflammatory drugs (OTC NSAIDS).

Compound	Cases	Controls	Multivariate OR[d] (95% CI)
None/Infrequent Use[a]	483	371	1.00
COX-2 Inhibitors[b]	13	61	0.15 (0.08-0.28)
Celecoxib	4	34	0.14 (0.05-0.43)
Rofecoxib	6	26	0.15 (0.06-0.37)
OTC NSAIDs[c]	91	162	0.43 (0.25-0.55)
Aspirin	67	109	0.46 (0.32-0.65)
Ibuprofen/Naproxen	24	53	0.36 (0.21-0.60)
Acetaminophen	24	21	0.98 (0.53-1.82)
Totals	611	615	

[a] No use of any NSAID or analgesic or infrequent use of no more than one pill per week for less than one year;

[b] COX-2 inhibitors include celecoxib, rofecoxib, valdecoxib, and meloxicam used daily for two years or more.

[c] Over the counter (OTC) NSAIDs/analgesics used at least two times per week for two years or more.

[d] Multivariate odds ratios are adjusted for continuous variables (age and body mass) and categorical variables (parity, menopausal status, family history, smoking, and alcohol intake).

Table 3 presents risk estimates for COX-2 inhibitors with stratification by menopause, family history, estrogen receptor and HER-2/*neu* status. The observed risk reductions were statistically significant and reasonable consistent across all strata. Cyclooxygenase-2 inhibitors produced significant risk reductions for premenopausal women (OR=0.12), postmenopausal women (OR=0.21), women with a positive family history (OR=0.19), women with a negative family history (OR=0.14), women with estrogen receptor positive tumors (OR=0.24), women with estrogen receptor negative tumors (OR=0.05), women with HER-2/neu positive tumors (OR=0.26), and women with HER-2/neu negative tumors (OR=0.17).

Table 3. Odds ratios for selective COX-2 inhibitors and breast cancer by strata of risk factors or cell membrane receptors.

Characteristic	Cases	Controls[a]	Multivariate OR[b] (95% CI)
Menopausal Status			
Premenopausal	251	289	0.12 (0.04-0.45)
Postmenopausal	360	326	0.21 (0.11-0.40)
Family History			
Positive	198	106	0.19 (0.06-0.56)
Negative	413	509	0.14 (0.06-0.30)
Estrogen Receptor			
Positive	226	--	0.24 (0.11-0.51)
Negative	71	--	0.05 (0.01-0.82)
HER-2/*neu*			
Positive	127	--	0.26 (0.06-0.72)
Negative	203	--	0.17 (0.07-0.44)

[a]Odds ratios for cell membrane receptor status (estrogen receptor and HER-2/neu) were calculated using the entire control group of women without breast cancer (n=615).
[b]Multivariate odds ratios are adjusted for continuous variables (age and body mass) and categorical variables (parity, menopausal status, family history, smoking, and alcohol intake).

Discussion

The results of this epidemiologic investigation reflect a significant risk reduction in human breast cancer due to intake of selective COX-2 inhibitors. Standard daily dosages of celecoxib (200 mg) or rofecoxib (25 mg) taken for two or more years were associated with an 85% reduction in breast cancer risk. Effects of the selective COX-2 inhibitors were consistent within subgroups of premenopausal and postmenopausal women, and women with and without a family history of breast cancer. Furthermore, risk reductions were also evident regardless of cell membrane receptors (estrogen receptors and HER-2/neu) measured at the time of diagnosis. Comparator NSAIDs with non-selective COX-2 activity (325 mg aspirin, 200 mg ibuprofen or 250 mg naproxen) also produced significant risk reductions, and it is notable that the effect of ibuprofen, a nonselective NSAID with significant COX-2 activity, was similar to that of selective COX-2 blocking agents. In contrast, acetaminophen did not change the risk of breast cancer.

In general, NSAIDs inhibit cyclooyxgenase which is the key rate-limiting enzyme of prostaglandin biosynthesis [15, 16, 17]. Molecular studies show that the inducible COX-2 gene is over-expressed in human breast cancer and that COX-2 genetic expression in cancer cells is correlated with mutagenesis, mitogenesis, angiogenesis, and deregulation of apoptosis [18, 19, 20]. Over the counter NSAIDs have consistently shown antitumor effects in animal models of carcinogenesis [21], and in recent studies, striking antitumor effects of the specific COX-2 inhibitor, celecoxib, have been observed against breast cancer [22]. In breast cancer cells, COX-2 over-expression is also associated with CYP-19 P-450$_{arom}$ genetic expression and local estrogen biosynthesis [23, 24, 25]. The current study coupled with existing preclinical and molecular evidence suggest that aberrant induction of COX-2 and upregulation of the prostaglandin cascade play a significant role in mammary carcinogenesis, and that blockade of this process has strong potential for intervention.

Enthusiasm for the use of selective COX-2 blocking agents in the chemoprevention of breast cancer and other malignancies has been tempered by reports of adverse effects on the cardiovascular system leading to the recall of popular anti-arthritic compounds, rofecoxib (Vioxx) and valdecoxib (Bextra). However, such studies involved supra-therapeutic dosages given over long periods of time without consideration of body size or individual differences in metabolism [26].

Conclusions

We observed a significant reduction in the risk of human breast cancer due to intake of selective COX-2 inhibitors. Chemopreventive effects against breast cancer were associated with recommended daily doses of celecoxib (median dose=200 mg) or rofecoxib (median dose=25 mg) for an average duration of 3.6 years. Notably, selective COX-2 inhibitors (celecoxib and rofecoxib) were only recently approved for use in 1999, and rofecoxib (Vioxx) was withdrawn from the marketplace in 2004. Nevertheless, even in the short window of exposure to these compounds, the selective COX-2 inhibitors produced a significant (85%) reduction in the risk of breast cancer, underscoring their strong potential for breast cancer chemoprevention.

Competing Interests

This research was supported in part by a grant from Pfizer, New York, NY, and grant P30 CA16058 from the National Cancer Institute, Bethesda, MD.

Author's Contributions

REH designed and directed the study. JBD coordinated data collection and quality control, and assisted in the interpretation of results. GAA assisted in the analysis and interpretation of results.

Acknowledgements

The authors thank Elvira M. Garofalo, Program Manager of the James Cancer Mammography Unit, and Julie M. Coursey, Assistant Director of the James Cancer Medical Records Registry, for their assistance in the conduct of this investigation.

References

[1]   Couzin J. Withdrawal of Vioxx casts a shadow over COX-2 inhibitors. *Science* 2004, 306, 384-385.

[2]   Couzin J. Clinical Trials: Nail-biting time for trials of drugs. Science 2004, 306, 1673-1675.

[3]   Mukherjee D, Nissen SE, Topol EJ. Risk of cardiovascular events associated with selective COX-2 inhibitors. J Am Med Assoc 2001, 286 (8): 954-959.

[4]   Bresalier RS, Sandler RS, Quan H, Bolognese JA, Oxenius B, Horgan K, Lines C, Riddell R, Morton D, Lanas A, Konstam MA, Baron JA. Cardiovascular events associated with rofecoxib in a colorectal adenoma chemoprevention trial. N Engl J Med 2005, 352 (11): 1092-1102.

[5]   Solomon SD, McMurray JJ, Pfeffer MA, Wittes J, Fowler R, Finn P, Anderson WF, Zauber A, Hawk E, Bertagnolli M. Cardiovascular risk associated with celecoxib in a clinical trial for colorectal adenoma prevention. N Engl J Med 2005, 352 (11), 1071-1080.

[6]   White WB, Faich G, Whelton A, Maurath C, Ridge NJ, Verburg KM, Geis GS, Lefkowith JB. Comparison of thromboembolic events in patients treated with celecoxib , a cyclooxygenase-2 specific inhibitor, versus ibuprofen or diclofenac. Am J Cardiol 2002, 89 (4): 425-430.

[7]   White WB, Faich G, Borer JS, Makuch RW. Cardiovascular thrombotic events in arthritis trials of the cyclooxygenase-2 inhibitor, celecoxib. Am J Cardiol 2003, 92 (4): 411-418.

[8]   Reicin AS, Shapiro D, Sperling RS, Barr E, Yu Q. Comparison of cardiovascular thrombotic events in patients with osteoarthritis treated with rofecoxib versus nonselective nonsteroidal anti-inflammatory drugs (ibuprofen, diclofenac, and nabumetone). Am J Cardiol 2002, 89 (2): 204-209.

[9]   Mamdani M, Rochon P, Juurlink DN, Anderson GM, Kopp A, Naglie G, Austin PC, Laupaci A. Effect of selective cyclooxygenase-2 inhibitors and naproxen on short-term risk of acute myocardial infarction in the elderly. Arch Intern Med 2003, 163 (4): 481-486.

[10]   Shaya FT, Blume SW, Blanchette CM, Weir MR, Mullin CD. Selective cyclooxygenase-2 inhibition and cardiovascular effects: an observational study of a Medicaid population. Arch Intern Med 2005, 165 (2): 181-186.

[11]   Cancer Statistics, Incidence and Mortality. American Cancer Society, 2004.

[12]   Harris RE, Beebe-Donk J, Doss H, Burr-Doss D. Aspirin, ibuprofen, and other non-steroidal anti-inflammatory drugs in cancer prevention: a critical review of non-selective COX-2 blockade (Review). Oncology Reports 2004, 13: 559-583.

[13]   Schlesselman JJ. Case Control Studies. Oxford University Press, New York, 1982.

[14]   Harrell F. Logistic Regression Procedure. Statistical Analysis System (SAS), 2005.

[15]   Vane JR. Inhibition of prostaglandin synthesis as a mechanism of action for aspirin-like drugs. *Nature* 1971, 231: 323-235.

[16]   Herschman HR. Regulation of prostaglandin synthase-1 and prostaglandin synthase-2. Cancer and Metas Rev 1994, 13: 241-256.

[17]   Hla T and Neilson K. Human cyclooxygenase-2 cDNA. Proc Natl Acad Sci USA 1992, 89: 7384-7388.

[18]   Harris RE. Epidemiology of breast cancer and nonsteroidal anti-inflammatory drugs. In: COX-2 Blockade in Cancer Prevention and Therapy, Edited by Harris RE. Humana Press, Totowa, NJ, 2002, 57-68.

[19]   Parrett ML, Harris RE, Joarder FS, Ross MS, Clausen KP, Robertson FM. Cyclooxygenase-2 gene expression in human breast cancer. International Journal of Oncology 1997, 10: 503-507.

[20]   Masferrer JL, Leahy KM, Koki AT, Aweifel BS, Settle SL, Woerner BM, Edwards DA, Flickinger AG, Moore RJ, Seibert K. Antiangiogenic and antitumor activities of cyclooxygenase-2 inhibitors. Cancer Res 2000, 60(5): 1306-1311.

[21]   Abou-Issa HM, Alshafie GA, Harris RE. Chemoprevention of breast cancer by nonsteroidal anti-inflammatory drugs and selective COX-2 blockade in animals. In: *COX-2 Blockade in Cancer Prevention and Therapy*, Edited by Harris RE. Humana Press, Totowa, NJ, 2002, 85-98.

[22]   Harris RE, Alshafie GA, Abou-Issa H, Seibert K. Chemoprevention of breast cancer in rats by Celecoxib, a specific cyclooygenase-2 (COX-2) inhibitor. *Cancer Res* 2000, 60: 2101-2103.

[23]   Harris RE, Robertson FM, Farrar WB, Brueggemeier RW. Genetic induction and upregulation of cyclooxygenase (COX) and aromatase (CYP-19): an extension of the dietary fat hypothesis of breast cancer. *Medical Hypotheses* 1999, 52 (4): 292-293.

[24]   Zhao Y, Agarwal VR, Mendelson CR, Simpson ER. Estrogen biosynthesis proximal to a breast tumor is stimulated by PGE2 via cyclic AMP, leading to activation of promoter II of the CYP19 (aromatase) gene. Endocrinology 1996, 137(12): 5739-5742.

[25]   Brueggemeier RW, Quinn AL, Parrett ML, Joarder FS, Harris RE, Robertson FM. Correlation of aromatase and cyclooxygenase gene expression in human breast cancer specimens. Cancer Letters l999, 140 (1-2):27-35.

[26]   Harris RE. Does the dose make the poison? Science 2005, 308, 203.

In: Cancer Prevention Research Trends
Editors: Louis Braun and Maximilian Lange

ISBN: 978-1-60456-639-0
© 2008 Nova Science Publishers, Inc.

Chapter VI

Counseling Undergraduates of the Health Care Professions in a Developing Country: Are there Peculiar Needs or Desires?

Olayinka. O. Omigbodun[1,*], *Akinyinka. O. Omigbodun*[2]
and Akin-Tunde A. Odukogbe[3]
[1]Senior Lecturer in Psychiatry,
[2]Professor of Obstetrics and Gynecology
[3]Sub-Dean (Undergraduate), Faculty of Clinical Sciences and Dentistry (2000-2002)
College of Medicine, University of Ibadan and University College Hospital,
Ibadan, Nigeria

Abstract

For many students, university life is extremely stressful. However studies suggest that undergraduates in the health care professions have peculiar stresses due to long hours of study and longer duration of study. Nigeria is a typical example of a developing country with all the problems of basic infrastructure. This implies that health care students may have to deal with stress not only from their course of study, but also from having to cope with living in a developing world context. Structured counseling services may help but are yet to be put in place. In developing counseling services, it is important to carry out a needs-assessment to identify what the students perceive their requirements to be.

This study utilizes both quantitative and qualitative methods to look into the circumstances the students recognize would require counseling, and also the type of facility desired. Having obtained informed consent from them, 1118 students of

* Address for Correspondence: Dr Olayinka Omigbodun, Department of Psychiatry, University College Hospital, Ibadan, Nigeria. Telephone: 234-2-2414102; Fax: 234-2-2413545; 4yinkas@skannet.com; fouryinkas@ yahoo.co.uk

medicine, dentistry, physiotherapy and nursing, completed questionnaires about their counseling needs and what they consider desirable in a counseling facility.

Twelve themes emerged as circumstances requiring counseling: academic problems, courtship and marriage issues, future career, financial problems, emotional problems, family problems, spiritual problems and issues of religion, problems with physical health, difficult teachers, problems with utilities (accommodation, transport, catering and related issues), sexual harassment, and alcohol/drug use.

Some of the conditions desired by the students for a counseling service were confidentiality, counselors with a 'good attitude', enlightenment campaigns, made optional for students, affordability and accessibility, and provision of a 24-hour service. Other features desired were a combined counseling service offered by professionals and lecturers, wide service coverage to include areas such as academic, emotional and spiritual counseling. There should also be sensitivity to ethnicity, culture and religious affiliation.

Undergraduates in their first year were more likely to request counseling for academic and emotional or psychological problems while students in their final year were more likely to request counseling about future careers and difficulty with teachers. Females were more likely to request counseling for academic problems while the males seemed to be more concerned with emotional and financial problems. The females required counseling as an avenue to ventilate and were particularly concerned about confidentiality while the males required it for decision making. Students showing evidence of psychological distress had a significantly different pattern of need for counseling in the areas of academic difficulties, emotional problems, finances and problems with utilities

The findings demonstrate that the counseling needs in these undergraduates are similar to what obtains in other parts of the world, although there are some needs, notably in the area of spiritual and religious issues, that derive from the developing country environment in which they are studying.

Introduction

For many students the passage into and coping with university life can be an extremely stressful and distressing experience (Rana, 2000). Several reasons may account for this. For some, it is the first time they have moved out of a secure home setting, with the impact of change and separation from two key supports, family and a familiar environment (Waller et al., 2005). Others need help coping with the tasks expected of them in the late adolescent period, identifying with other students, academic staff and the university at large, and if the move is into a big university, having to cope with the bureaucracy of a large organization (HUCS, 2002). Several studies on university students have found that if the stresses experienced in the course of pursuing a university education are left unchecked, this could have a detrimental effect on their mental health (Nolan and Wilson, 1994), academic output and consequent future prospects. One way to help the students cope with these changes is by providing on-going psychological support and counseling from the time of enrolment, and altering the content of this support to meet emergent needs until they graduate.

Situations Presenting for Counseling

Of great concern is the present suggestion from research studies that psychological distress is rampant and could be rising in incidence among university students (HUCS, 2002, Rana, 2000). Data from the Student Counseling Center at the University of Leeds show a rise in the number of clients each year between 1996 and 2003, and a rise in referrals to psychiatry much greater than the growth in the size of the population serving as the source of referral (Waller et al., 2005). Among University of Cambridge students in the UK, a fifth of the students reported at least one problem which caused them substantial worry, with academic problems causing the biggest concern, followed by financial issues and relationship problems (Surtees et al., 2000). Similarly there are suggestions that students presenting for counseling may have a higher risk of emotional, academic and financial problems (HUCS, 2002), a complex inter-relationship now recognized between these three factors and women found to be more distressed than men. This same study revealed that 10% of students had drug use problems and another 10% alcohol related problems. About 6% of women also reported eating disorders (Surtees et al, 2000). All these social and psychological factors are known to have a negative effect on academic outcome (Surtees et al., 2000).

In an assessment of the counseling facility at the University of Toronto, Canada (Coletti et al., 2005), mental health professionals who directly counsel students revealed that 30-40% of students who presented for counseling came for help with study skills and reported having high levels of stress. Mental health problems found among students presenting for counseling also included 25% diagnosed with depressive disorders, 10% with anxiety disorders and 5% with eating disorders. Mental health professionals also did not report any gender differences in stress levels but noted that women were more likely to seek help.

Stress among Students of Medicine and other Healthcare Professions

Over and above the well-documented stress associated with obtaining a university degree, it is generally believed that students in the health care professions experience even greater stress (Morrison, 2001; Jones and Johnston, 1997; Timmins and Kaliszer, 2002; Everly et al., 1994). This has stimulated an increase in research on stress and stress reduction in students of the health professions (Henning et al., 1998).

For medical students, there are suggestions that they face tremendous stress in the course of their study because the workload is heavier than for most other courses (Guthie et al., 1995; Supe, 1998). The course is also longer and hence more financially draining (Dangerfield, 2001). Some studies suggest that most stress occurs during the transition from preclinical to clinical training (Radcliffe and Lester, 2003; Helmers et al., 1997). Others suggest higher levels of stress in first year medical students due to the tremendous change in their lifestyle (Guthie et al., 1995; Lee and Graham, 2001). There are suggestions that up to a third of medical students may suffer from psychological morbidity as measured by the General Health Questionnaire (Guthie et al., 1995; Firth, 1986). In a similar fashion, dental students are also known to experience high levels of psychological stress (Sanders and

Lushington, 2002). A study of students in seven European dental schools indicated that 36% reported evidence of psychological morbidity, evidenced by a score of three or more on the General Health Questionnaire (Humphris et al., 2002)

According to Morrison (2001), the three major areas of stress for medical students are academic pressures, social pressures and financial problems. There are suggestions that factors causing stress may vary with the stage of training, with concerns about workload occurring mostly in the early stages (Guthie et al., 1995) and concerns about death, relationship with consultants and effects on personal life occurring in the later stages of training (Firth, 1986). Some of the stress experienced by medical and dental students found to be closely linked to psychological morbidity is 'student abuse' (Sheehan et al., 1990; Wolf et al, 1992).

Other studies suggest that high levels of stress and psychological morbidity are not limited to medical students but occur in students in other health care professions. Baccalaureate nursing students in Canada, regardless of year or university of attendance, experienced higher levels of stress, and higher levels of physiological and psychological symptoms than students in other health related disciplines (Beck et al., 1997), while distress, stress and coping in first year student nurses also exceeded levels in published studies of fourth year medical students and the general female population (Jones and Johnston, 1997). Also, a needs assessment of students in physical and occupational therapy programs in the United States of America identified stressors relating to the family, finances and adjustment to the student role as the key stress areas (Everly et al., 1994)

Use of Counseling Services

As a result of the now established evidence of the psychological pressures experienced by students in universities, most universities in the developed world have adopted a preventive approach to mental health and embedded counseling services into their systems. Unfortunately, research also suggests that not many students who would benefit from such services use it. In the University of Cambridge, 35% of students who reported having problems did not make use of available support facilities (Surtees et al., 2000). Only about 8% of students with problems approached the university's counseling service and these were students with very high levels of stress. However, those who used the counseling service benefited from this as 75% who used the service reported that help and advice given by the service helped to resolve their presenting problems (Surtees et al., 2000).

Several reasons have been found to be responsible for the reluctance of students to utilize counseling services (BACP, 2002; AUCC, 2001). These include the perceived stigma associated with seeking psychological help, lack of information about the service, misunderstanding of the service and preference for other help seeking behavior, which could be negative or positive.

Benefits of Counseling Services

Students who attended counseling were better equipped to attend to the challenges of university life, through better ability to cope, increased motivation, less likelihood of dropping out of school, and being better equipped to do their academic work (HUCS, 2002; Surtees et al., 2000; Caleb, 2002, Egert, 1999). In universities in the developed world, counseling provision can be described as well established in the university system (HUCS, 2002) with most universities having counseling programs in place. This is not the situation with several universities in developing countries many of whom are still battling with basic infrastructure and utility problems. Structured and well organized counseling services may not be priority despite the fact that several studies point to the effectiveness of counseling interventions in several aspects of university life.

Purpose of this Study

The authorities of the Faculty of Clinical Sciences and Dentistry at the University of Ibadan, Nigeria had recognized that there was a need for students in these extremely stressful courses to receive guidance and counseling. This recognition led to the establishment of a 'personal tutor support system, which entailed the allocation of 10 to 15 students randomly to each member of the academic staff who would serve as a 'staff advisor'. Informal observation and interviews with students and staff after the lists were released revealed that some students were happy with their randomly assigned personal tutor but many were not. Also several members of the Faculty were at a loss as regards what to offer the students allocated to them. Based on all these observed difficulties, the authors proceeded to design and carry out an assessment of the counseling needs of students in the Faculty, which could be used as a framework for designing a counseling service for students in the institution.

The specific objectives included the determination of the circumstances that the students thought would make them seek counseling, to ascertain what features the students would find desirable in a counseling service if one were established, and to ascertain the relationship between the presence of psychological distress and the students' perceived need for guidance and counseling.

Methodology

This study was conducted among the students of the University of Ibadan, Ibadan in Southwestern Nigeria. The University was the first one established in Nigeria. It was founded as a College of the University of London, United Kingdom in 1948 with three academic faculties, including a Faculty of Medicine, which was converted into a College of Medicine consisting of three faculties in 1980. One of those three faculties was the Faculty of Clinical Sciences and Dentistry, which consisted of Medical, Dental, Physiotherapy and Nursing students at the College of Medicine. [The Dental students are now in the Faculty of Dentistry, which was created in 2002].

All students in the Faculty of Clinical Sciences and Dentistry at the time of the study were the target population. Students in their preliminary year (100 Level) in the University were excluded from this study because this Level is a general introductory period of study where students take common courses before proceeding to their proposed course of study the following year at the 200 level. Some of the students bypass this preliminary year altogether by entering the university with Advanced Level certificates or a Diploma in Nursing.

With the preliminary year, the nursing and physiotherapy degree courses are four years in duration while dentistry and medicine are six years in duration. Both nursing and physiotherapy recently changed the duration of their program to five years. There is therefore a mixture of students from both the 4-year and 5-year nursing and physiotherapy programs among study participants. Data was collected in the month of July 2001.

Questionnaire

The questionnaire was anonymous and had a short consent form. Information on demographic details, sources of income and average monthly income were obtained. The students were also asked to rate their current financial situation on a scale of good, fair, difficult and desperate.

A question about the circumstances that might make the student seek guidance or counseling was then asked. They were also asked a question about whether or not they thought that counseling facilities could help alleviate their stress, with an option of writing a few statements explaining their 'Yes', 'No' or 'I don't know' responses. This qualitative method was included so that unknown themes could emerge from this group of students within this setting. They were also requested to make suggestions on what features they would like to see in a counseling service if one were provided, what sort of personnel should handle counseling and whether they would be prepared to pay for such a counseling service.

The last section of the questionnaire included the 12- item General Health Questionnaire (GHQ-12). The GHQ is a self-administered questionnaire designed to detect psychiatric disorders in community and other settings such as primary care (Goldberg and Williams, 1988). The GHQ-12 was chosen because it has been validated for use in this environment and is short and easy to complete, having only 12 items. The standard GHQ method of scoring 0-0-1-1 for each item was employed, which allows a maximum score of 12. In this study, three different cut-offs for the GHQ-12 are explored. These are scores of 1 & above, 2 & above and 3 & above. In a validity study of the GHQ-12 in this environment, the 1 & above cut-off was obtained as the optimum threshold with sensitivity of 77.8% and specificity of 79.4% (Gureje and Obikoya, 1990). In addition, this threshold allows for increased sensitivity and is suggestive of psychological distress. The higher cut-off points of 2 or more and 3 or more are also explored as they are more indicative of psychological disorder and allows for increased specificity.

Analysis

The researchers went through all the questionnaires to identify the various issues and circumstances the students felt would make them seek guidance/counseling. The answers given were grouped into themes, based on a qualitative analysis of the responses. The data were then entered and analyzed with the Statistical Package for the Social Sciences (SPSS version 10).

The data were analyzed quantitatively to determine the association between the individual thematic factors, identified in the qualitative analysis as those that would trigger off a request for counseling, and the socio-demographic characteristics of the students. An attempt was also made to ascertain any relationship between the student's perceived counseling needs and the presence of psychological morbidity as detected by the GHQ-12.

Statistical analysis was carried out using univariate analysis to relate each of the socio demographic factors and factors that would trigger a request for counseling, and to relate counseling needs to psychological distress detected by the GHQ-12. Variables showing significant associations during univariate analysis were then entered into stepwise multiple logistic regression models using the backward elimination method. Odds ratios and 95% confidence intervals (CI) associated with the various socio demographic variables relative to the factors that would make the student seek counseling were computed. This was also done for the GHQ score relative to the factors that would trigger a counseling request from the student. This method was used to determine the best-fit for socio-demographic variables that predict a need for counseling in specific areas of the students' lives, and also for assessing the impact of psychological distress on the perceived need for counseling on the part of the student.

Results

The target population for this study was all students in the Faculty of Clinical Sciences and Dentistry, which included medical, dental nursing and physiotherapy students. [The dental students are now in a new Faculty of Dentistry, created in 2002.] Out of the total number of 2093 students in the faculty at the time of the study, 1118 questionnaires were available for analysis, giving a response rate of 53%. Medical students had the lowest response rate with 847 out of 1683 (50.3%), followed by dental students with 116 out of 206 (56.3%), the physiotherapy students with 61% response (78 of 128) and the highest response rate of 100% coming from the 77 nursing students.

Socio-Demographic Characteristics of the Study Population

The socio demographic characteristics of the study population are summarized in Table 1. Over 70% of the students were aged 24 and below with a mean age of 23.71 (SD: 3.55). A higher proportion of female students than males completed the questionnaires when compared to the gender distribution in the target population, which was 58.7% male and 41.3% female. Most students (94.6%) were currently single, adding up those who described themselves as single, engaged or divorced. Christians constitute 90% of the population and the 1% described as others include religions like Eckankar, Grail Message, Lamaism and African traditional religions.

Nigeria is a country divided into the 36 states and a Federal capital territory. The country is also divided into 6 geopolitical zones, each consisting of five to eight states. The distribution of the students who participated in this study according their geopolitical zone of origin is also shown in Table 1. Over two-thirds of the students were from the Southwest zone where the university under study is situated, while the three geopolitical zones from the Northern part of the country had the lowest number, collectively contributing a total of only 6.9% of the students.

Table 1 . Socio Demographic Characteristics of the Study Population

Course	N (%)
Medicine	847 (76)
Dentistry	116 (10)
Physiotherapy	78 (7)
Nursing	77 (7)
Age (years)	
24 and below	759 (73)
25 to 30	237 (23)
31 and above	46 (4)
Gender	
Male	549 (51)
Female	529 (49)
Marital Status	
Single	958 (85.6)
Engaged	98 (8.8)
Married	49 (4.4)
Separated/Divorced	2 (0.2)
Religion	
Islam	100 (9)
Christian Orthodox	329 (30)
Christian Pentecostal	665 (60)
Other Religions	11 (1)
Course Level	
200	147 (13)
300	293 (26)
400	370 (33)
500	155 (14)
600	152 (14

Course	N (%)
Geopolitical Regions of Origin	
Southwest	747 (67.8)
Southeast	117 (10.6)
Southsouth	162 (14.7)
Northwest	3 (0.3)
Northeast	3 (0.3)
Northcentral	69 (6.3)

What Problems/Circumstances Might Make Students Require Guidance or Counseling?

In a qualitative analysis of the responses, twelve themes emerged as circumstances that the students considered would make them seek counseling and they are shown in Table 2. Counseling for academic issues was the most frequent request (44.4%), followed by future career guidance (17.4%) and financial issues (16.1%). Sexual harassment and drug/alcohol use or abuse both tied for last place (0.4%) among the reasons the students considered as likely to make them seek counseling.

Table 2. Students' perception of the circumstances that might make them seek counseling

Issues Requiring Counseling	N (%)
Academic Problems	496 (44.4)
Courtship/Marriage/Love-life/Relationship Problems	245 (21.9)
Guidance for Future Career	194 (17.4)
Financial Guidance	180 (16.1)
Emotional Problems	166 (14.8)
Family Problems	60 (5.4)
Spiritual and Religious Issues	57 (5.1)
Health Problems	50 (4.5)
Difficulty With Teachers	50 (4.5)
Utilities and Transportation Issues	33 (3.0)
Sexual Harassment	4 (0.4)
Issues Relating to Drug and Alcohol Use	5 (0.4)

The range of views and examples of the students' requests from which these 12 themes were drawn are displayed in Text Boxes 1 – 12 below:

Text Box 1.

Academic Issues

'Poor and un-improving academic performance'
'Study plan'
'Not doing well in class tests'
'They have to examine why one scores very low marks after we have prepared very well'
'Studying techniques'
'How to overcome [the subject of] surgery?'
'How to remember enough to pass?'
'Irregularity with academic program'
'Study guidance'
'Coping with work load'
'Failure of tests and examinations'
'Stressful surgery postings and [attendance] booklets that are too difficult to fill'
'Time management'
'Dwindling interest in medicine'
'How to write essays'
'Strategies on reading and assimilation'
'Best way to end up with distinction in all my clinical postings'
'The attitude of doctors to medical students and their disrespect'
'I don't understand biochemistry at all and, being off campus, I don't attend discussion classes'
'The lecturers are so fast I don't understand anything in the lecture room unless I read by myself'
'How to combine extracurricular activities with academic work'

Text Box 3.

Guidance for Future Career

'Deciding what specialty to do'
'Choice of career'
'What next after medical school?'
'Getting a space for house job here'
'Life after school'
'When considering area of specialty in the future'
'Career prospect in physiotherapy'
'Future as a medical doctor and options available for specialization'
'How will employment be available in Nigeria?'
'Whether to change career'

Text Box 2.

Relationships/Courtship/Marriage/Love-life

'Marital counseling'
'Choice of spouse'
'Stress from lover'
'Relationship with opposite sex'
'Relationship with people around'
'Dating'
'Difficult times in my relationship'
'Dealing with people'
'Marriage problems'
'Boy/girls'
'Courtship'
'Too many girlfriends'
'When I feel cheated by my colleagues'
'Death of loved ones'

Text Box 4.

Financial Guidance

'Inadequate money'
'An income as a medical student'
'Financial crisis'
'Income management'
'Getting financial aid and scholarships'
'How to make money quickly'
'Discipline in spending'

Table 6.

Family Problems

'Parents' induced stress'
'Recovering from my mothers death'
'When offended by my parents'
'I feel unloved especially by my mother'
'Family pressure'
'Family instability'
'Being compared to other members who
    studied medicine'
'Parent's interference in choice of course'
'If I were to have a family problem'
'Family problems'

Text Box 5.

Emotional Issues

'Disallowing emotional situations from
    perturbing my psyche'
'Depression'
'Unexplained sadness'
'Depression due to overstaying [in school]'
'Lack of concentration'
'Motivation'
'Making up my own mind'
'How to enjoy life'
'The fact that my mates outside are moving
    forward either in academics or work and here
    I feel stagnant'
'Facing a crowd or gathering'
'Anxiety'
'Losing confidence'
'Bad thoughts'
'Confusion'
'Fear'
'Identity problems'
'Loneliness'
'Lack of confidence and timidity'
'When I am angry, I can't even hide it'
'I don't trust at all'
'Relieving tension'
'Fear of disease, e.g. HIV, in the line of study'

Text Box 7.

Spiritual and Religious Issues

Combining spiritual matters with profession
Christian life
Spiritual issues
Religions problems
Difficulties in hearing God
Difficulty in knowing the power of Jesus
    resurrection
Difficulty in obeying God
Difficulty in experiencing the cross
Difficulty in understanding God
Religions (Lack of belief)
Backsliding

Text Box 8.

Health Problems

'Health problems'
'Non-specific symptoms of illness'
'During uncertainty of illness'
'Physical health'
'General feeling of being unwell'
'Weight problem'

Text Box 9.

Difficulty with Teachers and Authorities

'Problems with certain teachers'
'Victimization by teachers'
'Insults by lecturers'
'Right to say and put forward opinion about lecturers'
'How to handle disappointment by lecturers and
    heads of departments who shift graduation dates;
    its so frustrating and a very sad thing to be
    happening in the 21st century'
'Abuses by doctors on ward rounds as if there is
    something wrong with your head'
'The gap between students and doctors'
'Lecturer-student relationship'
'Fear of nasty consultants [Attending Specialists]'

Text Box 10.

Utilities and Transportation Issues

Accommodation
Lack of recreational facilities
Provision of facilities in the hall
Insecurity and crime wave in the halls of
    residence
The accommodation strain
Transportation costs
Feeding arrangements
Lack of water supply
Inconsistency of electricity supply

Text Box 11.

Sexual Harassment
'Sexual harassment by Lecturers'

Text Box 12.

Issues Relating to Drug and Alcohol Use
'Smoking and drinking'
'Drug abuse'

Association between Factors Triggering Counseling Requests and the Socio-Demographic Characteristics of the Respondents

Each factor that respondents identified as being likely to motivate a request for counseling was then looked at in relation to the socio-demographic characteristics such as age, gender, marital status, religion, geopolitical region of origin, level of study in the University, course of study, employment situation, place of residence, and financial situation.

Academic Issues

On univariate analysis, 4 socio-demographic attributes were related to a request for academic counseling: gender, region of origin, level of study and course of study.

Gender

More females requested for academic counseling, 48.5% females as opposed to 41% males ($\chi^2 = 6.12$; df: 2; $p = 0.013$).

Region of Origin

Students from the Southwest geopolitical zone of the country were the least likely to request for academic counseling. The proportion of students from each zone who would request for counseling are Southwest: 41.9%, Southeast: 54.7%, South-south: 48.8% and North: 45.3% respectively ($\chi^2 = 8.18$; df: 3; $p = 0.042$)

Level of Study

The greatest demand for academic counseling was in the first year of study. The specific proportions from each of the levels in the university were 200 Level: 55.8%; 300 Level: 46%; 400 Level: 43.9%; 500 Level: 41.3% and 600 Level: 41.4% ($\chi^2 = 9.58$; df: 4; $p = 0.048$)

Course of Study

Nursing students made the most requests for academic counseling, while the least requests came from the physiotherapy students. Among each student group, the proportions requiring counseling were Medicine: 44.4%; Dentistry: 41.4%; Physiotherapy: 34.6% and Nursing: 58.4% ($\chi^2 = 9.6$; $p = 0.022$)

When all of these factors were entered into a logistic regression equation, gender, region of origin and level of study were the three factors found to be strongly and independently associated with a request for academic counseling as shown in Table 3. The odds that a student will not require academic counseling rises with the level of study, a trend that is clearly shown in Figure 1.

Relationships, Courtship and Marriage Issues

None of the socio-demographic attributes studied was significantly associated with a request for counseling concerning relationships, courtship and marriage.

Future Career

Univariate analysis revealed age, level of study in the university and gender as the 3 factors that were significantly associated with a request for counseling concerning future careers.

Age

The much older as well as the very young students were the least likely to request counseling on future career choices. The percentage of students requesting counseling in each of the age groups were 15.7% of those 24years and under, 25.3% of those aged 25 to 30 and 6.5% of those aged 31 and above ($\chi^2 = 15.58$; df: 2; $p < 0.001$).

Level of Study

With increasing level of study, the requests for future career counseling increased thus: 200 Level: 3.4%; 300 Level: 10.6%; 400 Level: 16.3%; 500 Level: 27.1% and 600 Level: 36.2%. ($\chi^2 = 77.69$; df: 4; $p < 0.001$)

Course of Study

The medical and dental students were more likely to request for future career counseling than the physiotherapy and student nurses as demonstrated by the percentage in each group that would make the request – Medical: 19.4%; Dental: 15.5%; Physiotherapy: 11.5%; Nursing: 3.9%. (χ^2 = 14.21; df:3; p = 0.003).

After logistic regression, only the course and level of study were retained as factors significantly associated with counseling need in this area. Medical and dental students required this service the most; in fact medical students were 14 times more likely to require this kind of service compared with the Nursing students (See Table 3). The chances of a student requiring counseling about future career choices rose steadily with increasing level of study as seen in Figure 1.

Financial Counseling

On univariate analysis, older students, males and those reporting financial difficulty were more likely to request for financial counseling.

Age

The proportions requiring the service were 13.2% of those aged 24 and below, 20.7% of students between 25 and 30years and 26.1% of those aged 31years and above (χ^2 = 11.88; df: 2 p = 0.003).

Gender

Among the male students 19.5% needed counseling in this area, compared to 12.7% of their female counterparts (χ^2 = 9.18; df: 1; p = 0.002).

Reported Financial Situation

Among the students who reported good or fair finances 13.3% would request financial counseling, compared to 39.1% of those who reported difficult or desperate finances (χ^2 = 56.53; df: 1; p < 0.001). After logistic regression, financial situation and age were retained as significant factors predicting a need for the service (Table 3).

Table 3.Odds Ratios and 95% Confidence Intervals for Association of Counseling Requests With Socio-Demographic Factors After Logistic Regression

Socio-Demographic Factors	Areas of Request for Counseling				
	Academic Problems	*Future Career*	*Family Problems*	*Emotional Problems*	*Financial Issues*
	Odds Ratios and (95% Confidence Intervals)				
Gender	0.709 (0.55-0.91)			0.656 (0.46-0.93)	
Age					1.498 (1.12-1.99)

Region	0.863 (0.76-0.98)				
Course (Compared To Nursing)					
Medicine		14.862 (2.05-107.94)	0.366 (0.170-0.787)		
Dentistry		10.944 (1.41-84.86)			
Physiotherapy			0.198 (0.041-0.951)		
Level Of Study (Compared To 200-Level)					
300	1.672 (1.104-2.533)	3.524 (1.328-9.351)		0.567 (0.34-0.95)	
400	1.692 (1.134-2.527)	6.127 (2.382-15.758)		0.545 (0.33-0.89)	
500	1.767 (1.104-2.829)	9.438 (3.587-24.835)		0.43 (0.23-0.80)	
600	1.812 (1.133-2.899)	14.095 (5.414-36.699)		0.27 (0.13-0.54)	
Reported Financial Situation					4.161 (1.12-1.99)

Emotional Problems

Gender, level of study and reported financial situation were the three characteristics significantly associated with a request for counseling related to emotional issues and problems.

Gender
Males (17.7%) were more likely than females (12.3%) to request for emotional counseling ($\chi^2 = 6.04$; df: 1; $p = 0.014$)

Level of Study
Students in their first year of study were also more likely to request for emotional counseling compared to students in their latter years of study as shown by the proportion at each level that would request for help in this area: 200 Level (25.2%); 300 Level (15.0%); 400 Level (14.6%); 500 Level (12.3%) and 600 Level (7.9%) [$\chi^2 = 19.01$; df: 4; $p = 0.001$].

Financial Situation
Students who reported a difficult or desperate financial situation (21.1%)were more likely to request for emotional counseling compared to 13.7% of those who reported a good or fair situation ($\chi^2 = 5.03$; df: 1; $p = 0.025$)

Upon logistic regression, gender and level of study were strongly and independently associated with a request for counseling for emotional issues. There was a trend toward a decline in the need for emotional counseling with increasing level of study as demonstrated clearly in Figure 1.

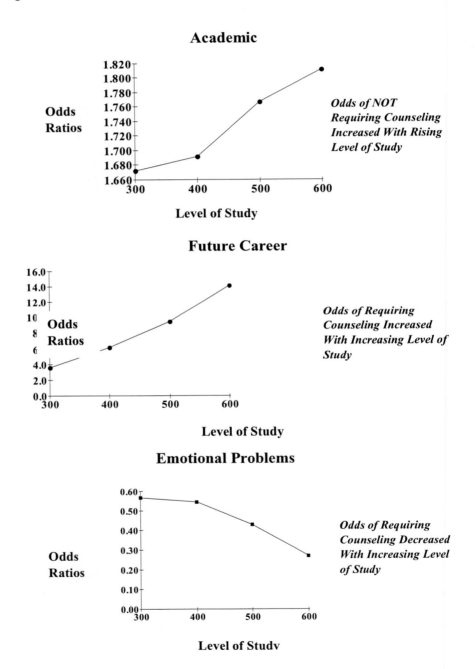

Figure 1. Relationship of level of study with need for counseling on academic issues, future career and emotional problems.

Family Problems

On univariate analysis, marital status and course of study were the two characteristics that were significantly associated with a request for counseling about family problems.

Marital Status

Among those who would request for counseling for family problems, 5.1% were single and 12.2% married ($\chi^2 = 4.65$; df: 1; $p = 0.031$)

Course of Study

The proportions that would request counseling on family problems from each course of study were Medicine: 4.7%; Dentistry: 7.8%; Physiotherapy: 2.6% and Nursing: 11.7% ($\chi^2 = 9.26$; df: 3; $p = 0.026$)

After logistic regression, course of study was the only factor that was retained as significant, with students of Medicine and Physiotherapy much less likely to need counseling than those of Dentistry and Nursing (Table 3).

Spiritual Problems and Issues of Religion

No socio demographic attributes were associated with a request for spiritual counseling.

Health Problems

None of the socio-demographic factors was significantly associated with a request for counseling about health problems.

Difficulty with Teachers

On doing univariate analysis, the age of the students and the level of study were the two socio-demographic factors that were significantly related to a counseling need for difficulty with teachers.

Age

Students who were 31years or more did not request for counseling for difficulty with teachers at all while 4% of those aged 24 years or less and 7.2% of those aged 25-30years made a request for the service ($\chi^2 = 6.605$; $p = 0.037$)

Level of Study

The final year students made the greatest request for counseling for difficult teachers. The proportions at each level of study were 200 Level: 3.4%; 300 Level: 2%; 400 Level: 5.7%; 500 Level: 2.6% and 600 Level: 9.2% ($\chi^2 = 14.96$; df: 4; $p = 0.005$)

On logistic regression however, neither of these two factors was retained as being significant.

Accommodation, Transportation and Other Utilities

None of the socio-demographic factors was associated with a request for counseling in this area.

Sexual Harassment

Only females (0.8%) requested counseling for sexual harassment but the proportion was so low as not to reach the level of statistical significance. ($p = 0.057$ [Fishers exact test]).

Drug and Alcohol Problems

The number of students requesting for counseling for drugs and alcohol were very few. No student from the Northern geopolitical zones made a request for drug and alcohol counseling compared to 0.1% of students from the South-west, 0.9% of those from the South-east and 1.9% of students from the South-south 1.9%, a significant difference ($p = 0.024$).

Summary of Attributes Independently Associated with a Need for Counseling

Table 3 summarizes the factors that were retained as being strongly and independently associated with need in the different areas of counseling, after logistic regression analysis. Male students were less likely to request for academic counseling while female students were less likely to request for emotional counseling. The only area of counseling where age is an independently associated factor is that of financial counseling with persons aged 31 years and above more likely to request the service.

Students from the Southwest geopolitical zone were the least likely to request for academic counseling. A look at the course of study reveal that students of Medicine were 14.8 times, and those of Dentistry 10.9 times more likely to request future career counseling compared to Nursing students. Medical and physiotherapy students were also less likely to request counseling for family issues. All other years of study except the first year or 200 Level were less likely to request counseling for emotional issues. The other factor strongly and independently associated with a request for financial counseling was reporting difficult and desperate finances.

Counseling Needs and Psychological Distress

The General Health Questionnaire findings will be examined at three different cut off points. Using a cut off of 3 or more, 250 (23.4%) had evidence of psychological distress, 403 (36%) of the students scored 2 or more on the GHQ, while 593 (53%) scored one or more.

Counseling requests were also looked at in relation to the GHQ scores. Univariate analysis revealed 7 areas where the students showing evidence of psychological distress were significantly more likely to request being counseled when related to the different GHQ scores. These are academic issues, relationship and marital issues, emotional problems, physical health problems, spiritual problems, financial problem and problems related to accommodation and utilities. These are shown in Table 4.

Table 4. Relationship Between Psychological Morbidity and Counseling Requests

GHQ at the 3 different cut-offs	Academic	Relationships	Emotional	Health	Spiritual	Financial	Utilities
	p-values						
GHQ 3 or more	0.005	0.037	<0.001		0.017	<0.001	0.004
GHQ 2 or more	0.004		0.001	0.026		<0.001	0.002
GHQ 1 or more	0.001		<0.001		0.027	0.004	0.034

**Table 5. Counseling Requests and Psychological Distress
(Odds Ratios and 95% Confidence Intervals After Logistic Regression)**

GHQ at the 3 different cut-offs	Academic	Emotional	Financial	Utilities
GHQ 3 or more	1.349 (1.01-1.81)	0.352 (0.35-0.73)	0.384 (0.38-0.79)	0.187 (0.19-0.82)
GHQ 2 or more	1.32 (1.02-1.71)	0.586 (0.42-0.83)	0.610 (0.43-0.85)	0.34 (0.16-0.74)
GHQ 1 or more	1.411 (1.09-1.82)	0.473 (0.33-0.69)	0.691 (0.49-0.98)	

After logistic regression, the areas where areas of requests for counseling were strongly and independently associated with psychological illness or distress at the three different GHQ scores are seen in Table 5. A request for academic, emotional and financial counseling were strongly and independently associated with psychological morbidity at the three different cutoff points.

Need For Counseling Facilities

In assessing the students' perception as to whether a counseling service could help them cope with stress and what they would need in such a counseling service, they gave the following responses to the questions posed to them.

Will Guidance and Counseling Facilities Help to Alleviate Your Stress?

A large plurality of the respondents (47.4%) were of the opinion that counseling facilities will help to alleviate their stress, as the pie chart in Figure 2 shows.

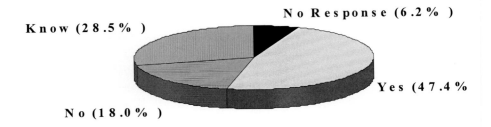

Figure 2. Role For Counseling in Alleviating Stress.

Of the 528 respondents who gave a 'yes' reply to the question that counseling would help to alleviate their stress, 410 went on to give a description on why they felt the counseling facilities would help.

Three themes emerged from the answers they provided on why counseling facilities would be helpful. These themes are shown in Table 6.

Table 6. Why Counseling Services Are Needed (N = 410)

		N (%)
	Will be Able to Ventilate/It Provides Some Relief	191 (46.4)
1.	'Because it will afford me the opportunity to talk about it and that in itself is medicine'	
2.	'Just talking to someone sometimes is very soothing'	
3.	'Pouring out ones soul is therapeutic'	
4.	'A problem shared is half solved'	
5.	'At times, discussing issues makes you feel better'	
6.	'Having someone that would listen to me would go a long way'	
	Information Given Will Help to Make the Right Decisions	174 (42.4)
1.	'Adequate information and guidance can help one to make the right decisions on what to specialize in, which determines one's future happiness'	
2.	'One can get advice on how to solve the problem'	
3.	'Allows sharing your problems with older and wiser person who would proffer some solution'	
4.	'It will help me in making decisions faster'	
5.	'You are able to talk to someone who has gone through the system and survived, so this could be encouraging and the person could offer practical tips	
6.	'Some tips can be given - relevant advice that can help me'	
	Counselors can Give Feedback to the Authorities	45 (11.2)
1.	'The counselors can feedback to the school authority'	
2.	'Maybe talking to a surgeon would make them take things easy with us. Maybe our teachers would be more democratic and less autocratic in decision making concerning our lives'	
3.	'I will be able to communicate with the authority through the counselor'	
4.	'The administration will get better feedback from students'	
5.	'Through this the counselor can appreciate our problems and suggest changes at a higher level'	

These three themes were analyzed in relationship to the different socio-demographic factors of the respondents and only gender showed a significant relationship.

Gender and Reasons Given for Why Counseling is Needed

The female students were more likely to mention 'a need to ventilate' (females 53.8%; males 39.4%) while more of the male students requested 'information to make decisions' (males 49.5%, females 35.0%). Both groups requested for 'feedback to authorities' in about equal proportions: 10.8% of males and 11.2% of females (χ^2 = 9.5; df: 2; p = 0.008).

Why Counseling Will Not Alleviate Stress

Of the 200 students who opined that counseling would not help them, 146 gave specific reasons why they held that opinion. Three themes emerged from the reasons given, as seen in Table 7.

Table 7. Why Counseling Services are not needed (N=146)

	N (%)
Counseling cannot help my stress areas such as money, infrastructure and utilities 1. 'They cannot provide recreational facilities or help with my health problems and most lecturers are lord's unto themselves' 2. 'Because I do not think the problem is basically mine' 3. 'I'm as good as out of the system now, even if I were still to be in, I would prefer that I am given a room to myself and money that I can use rather than counseling' 4. 'I can't discuss personal non-academic problems with a counselor, can a counselor give me a holiday' 5. 'There is nothing counseling can do about electricity supply' 6. 'The stress is man-made. The system needs overhauling'	109 (74.7)
Counseling should be given to the lecturers instead 1. 'The problem is with the professors. They are not trained to be lecturers, they need a diploma in education' 2. 'Lecturers themselves need counseling' 3. 'I don't know but I think it is our lecturers who need counseling'	10 (6.8)
I can take care of myself 1. 'Over the years I have learnt to adapt rapidly to any situation that arises' 2. 'I believe in myself' 3. 'I have always managed well without any external counseling, God is my counselor' 4. 'Because I have got to the stage were I can solve my own problems'	27 (18.5)

When the three reasons given for why counseling may not be useful to them were analyzed relative to the respondents' socio-demographic characteristics, there was a significant relationship with the age of the students. Students who were 25 years and above were more likely to report that they do not need counseling because they can take care of themselves (33.3%), compared to only 12.9% of those aged 24 years and below. Older students (> 25 years old) were more likely to report that the lecturers needed help (10.3%) compared to 4% among those aged 24 years and below. However the younger students were more likely to mention that the stress was coming from areas not amenable to counseling (83.2%) compared to 56.4% among those 25 years or older (χ^2 = 10.96; p = 0004).

Should Lecturers Provide Counseling?

The students were asked specifically if they would like their lecturers to provide the counseling. The pie chart in Figure 3 reveals that only about one-third of the students wanted their lecturers to provide the counseling and nearly 40% do not like the idea.

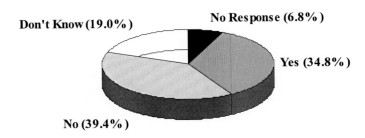

Figure 3. Should Lecturers be the Counselors?

Among the students who wanted their lecturers to provide the counseling service, five themes emerged from the reasons they provided for favoring that approach, after qualitative analysis as seen in Text Box 13, while Text Box 14 displays the eight themes derived from the responses of those providing reasons why lecturers should not provide counseling.

Text Box 13. Reasons Why Lecturers Should Provide Counseling
Lecturers have been in a similar situation before 'They probably have an idea of what I am going through and might have solutions' 'They have passed through similar stress before' 'Would prefer the lecturers because they have been through the system and some are close to us and can be quite fatherly or motherly amongst other reasons' 'Most if not all have been through the same things, so they can be of help more effectively' 'Yes, but not all the lecturers. Some of them are really mothers and fathers and since they are in the medical field, they understand peculiar problems. NB NOT ALL OF THEM ARE FIT FOR SUCH DUTIES!' 'They were once students' 'Because they know the rigor one is passing through in the nursing department'
Knowledge of students' problems will reflect in their attitude to teaching 'It helps the lecturers to improve in the approach to lecturing. So they don't just think we should be able to cope.' 'They can identify our limitations and it helps to know that they understand what we are going through' 'They will know our problems and this will reflect in their attitude towards us and their manner of teaching'
Lecturers are good if they receive training 'You see, our lecturers are not teachers—they are doctors, nothing more nothing less. That you have FRCS, FWACS (What have you) does not make you a teacher—College of Medicine should know this by now. If our lecturers are so trained, that is in counseling, why not? But in their present state, they need a lot of counseling themselves'

Lecturers are good but for academic and career counseling only
'I prefer interaction with them to be strictly for academics'
'Because most of my problems are school oriented they will know better'
'Lecturers will be able to counsel effectively in the academic area'
'For the counseling I have in mind the lecturers know better about residency programs than anyone else'
'On issues that may be career linked'
Will enhance a good student-lecturer relationship
'It will help them too to know what complaints the students have against them'
'It could bring a sort of closeness between the students and lecturers'

Text Box 14.
Reasons Why Lecturers Should Not Provide Counseling

Lecturers are not sensitive to students needs/unapproachable
'I really do not trust them, one minute they are nice and the next they are terrifying'
'Because they form the policies with which the school is required to run and some of these policies constitute our real and perceived problems.'
'Some are not approachable'
'Most students see their lecturers as being so high and mighty and feel they cannot relate to them'
'A master servant relationship is what obtains in the majority of cases'
'Poor relationship in quite a number of instances, few father and mother figures identified'
'Majority are incapable of counseling anybody by virtue of the fact the they have a role to play in the genesis of the problem'
'How can a problem be the solution'

Will affect interpersonal relationships with lecturers
'When your secrets are in someone's cupboard and you keep seeing the person daily, you will start feeling somehow'
'It may affect interpersonal relationships later'

Lecturers are equally stressed and project their frustrations
'Many of them are equally stressed. Some even project their frustrations on us.'

Lecturers are not skilled for counseling
'It should be the job of a skilled psychologist'
'They are not professional counselors'
'They may not be suitable qualified as counselor though they are lecturers'
'They are not trained to counsel'
'I do not think they are equipped to do it, counseling is not just being a good surgeon'

Need a neutral person
'Because I will not feel free to talk to them'
'I think it will be easier to tell my problems to someone I do not know'
'I would be free with people I don't see everyday or who I don't have to face many times after exposing myself'
'An unbiased person is always suitable'

Fear of victimization
'Because they might not be able to separate my personal life from my academic life, might use it as a weapon to victimize me'
'They might become vindictive'
'They can use it against you'

Will create unnecessary emotional attachments
'It could breed intimacy'
'Because relationships between students and lecturers should be kept strictly formal and some lecturers would not be able to remain detached and professional'

Lecturers will not have time
'They will not have enough time'

Type of Facility Desired

The bar chart in Figure 4 reveals the features desired by the students in a counseling facility that would be provided for them.

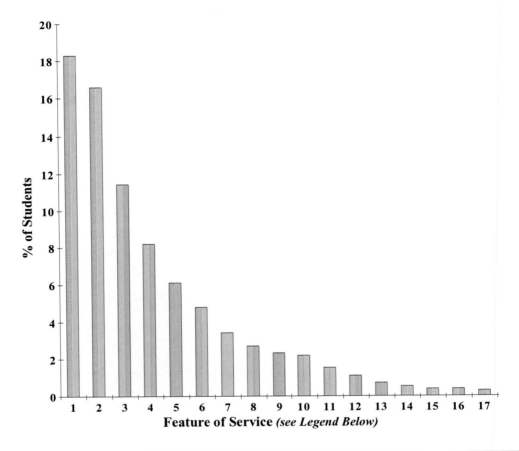

Legend to the x-axis (*Feature of Service*)		
1 Good Attitude	7 Involve Users	13 Optional for Students
2 Confidentiality	8 Sensitive to Ethnicity/ Culture/Religion	14 Identify Academically Weak Students
3 Affordable/Accessible 24/7	9 Enlightenment Campaigns on Use	15 Website (Anonymous) Service
4 Professional Counselors	10 Trained Lecturers	16 Group Counseling
5 Wide Range of Services	11 Monitor & Evaluate	17 Lecturers only to Provide Service
6 One-to-One Service	12 Combined Service (Lecturers & Professionals)	

Figure 4. Features That Should be Present in the Counseling Facility to be Provided A qualitative analysis of the description given by the students from which these themes of the type of counseling facility that they would prefer were derived is provided in Text Box 15.

Text Box 15.
Analysis of the Description of Features Desired by the Students in
a Counseling Facility

Confidentiality /Located Discreetly
Ensure confidentiality / Make sure there is privacy and secrecy
Comfortable and private venue
Assurance that what I say will not be used against me
Should be situated away from the hall of residence, but accessible
Good Attitude/ Cheerful Counselors/ Proven Character, Friendly Atmosphere, God Fearing
Ensure people who are appointed be of proven character (moral and spiritual) preferably happily married men and women
Select trustworthy and married adults as counselors
Friendliness and hospitality
Choose people who are approachable and student friendly
Identify academically weak students and invite for counseling
Monitor & evaluate – feedback to authorities to make improvements
Records should be kept and analyzed. Analysis and deduction be made available to the school authority for action about it
Feedback from the beneficiaries is very important
Regular review to see if it achieves its aims and objectives of being set up
Affordable/Accessible/24 hr service
Operate an open door policy
Counselors must be accessible, even after working hours
Affordable, Freely accessible
The service should be made free for all students
A nice environment with counselors on duty throughout the day
If have to choose lecturers – Select appropriate ones/Students choose/ with high moral standards/ give refresher course
To involve only lecturers that believe in the need for such facilities
Not every lecturer is fit to b a counselor as some of these lecturers instill mortal fear in students. Hence for anybody setting up this facility try to assess the lecturers and those who are friendly, understanding, reasonable who have the time should be chosen for such and not lecturers students will rather not have anything to do with.
One-to-one service
Person to person counseling / One-on-one counseling
One on one interactive session between the student and counselor that will span over a considerable period of time
Private person to person discussion
I would like a face to face meeting with the counselor and I would like to be the only one with her or him
Professional/ Trained Counselors
A separate facility with professionals
Preferably professional counselors should be used
Counselors should have undergo at least 4 months intensive training preferably in the United States
Should have basic education in counseling
Set up a standard counseling service with professionals in that field
I will prefer a guidance and counseling facility offered by a well meaning psychiatrist or clinical psychologist
Combined service with professionals and lecturers
Preferably professional counselors and genuinely interested lecturers
Counseling on the Internet
Website for anonymous counseling: A website where you can access any lecturers you choose and communicate without them necessarily knowing your true identity until you so choose

Text Box 15. (Continued)
Offer wide services such as academic/emotional/spiritual counseling, Have counselors with different areas of specialization Pre-entry counseling before decision to study medicine is made How to cope to with academics, spiritual growth and relationships Student should be referred to specialist in area of problem Know the principle of time management One which has specific people for different problems as they can be very good at what they do
Sensitivity to ethnic, culture/ belief systems/religious beliefs No religious sentiments To suit the peculiar nature of our culture and beliefs so as to make it feasible and long-lasting Let the composition of the team cut across all ethnic groups They must bear in mind the cultural and religious diversity of Nigeria
Involve Users, Free to change Counselor if need be, Let Users Choose Take an opinion from the population the facility is to cater for Involvement of the people who are to use the service Encourage student participation at all stages Make provisions to be able to change ones counselor Let students choose their own counselors
Lecturers only To involve only lecturers that see the need for such a facility/ Senior consultants should be selected first
Group Counseling Make it a group discussion. Ensure Small groups

Would you be willing to pay for a Counseling Facility?

The chart in Figure 5 shows that only about a quarter of the students would be willing to pay for a counseling service if one were to be provided.

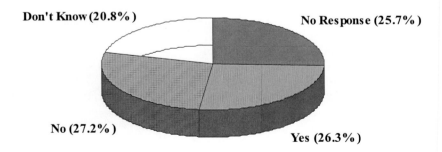

Figure 5. Willingness to Pay for Counseling Services.

The students who gave a yes or no answer to whether they would pay for a counseling service were then analyzed in relationship to their socio-demographic characteristics. On univariate analysis, three factors were significantly associated with willingness to pay for a counseling service, gender, course of study and reported financial situation.

Gender

Among the females 55.4% were willing to pay for a counseling service compared to 46.6% of the males ($\chi^2 = 4.48$; df: 1; $p = 0.034$).

Course of Study

The nursing students (63.2%) were the most willing to pay followed by the dental (51.7%) and medical students (51.5%) and the least likely to want to pay were the physiotherapy students (30.8%) ($\chi^2 = 11.94$; df: 3; $p = 0.008$).

Reported Financial Situation

Students most willing to pay for this service reported good finances (59.7%), followed by fair (49.7%), difficult (43.3%) and desperate finances (26.7%) [$\chi^2 = 9.5$; $p = 0.022$].

Following logistic regression, the two factors retained are course of study and financial situation as seen in Table 8. Medical and physiotherapy students were least likely to be willing to pay for a counseling service and students who report good finances are strongly and independently associated with willingness to pay to a counseling service.

Table 8. Odds Ratios and 95% Confidence Intervals of the Association Between Socio-Demographic Factors and Willingness to Pay For a Counseling Service

Socio-Demographic Factor	Odds Ratio	95% CI	p
Course			
Medicine	0.500	0.273-0.916	0.025
Physiotherapy	0.211	0.090-0.495	< 0.001
Reported Finances			
Good	2.082	1.105-3.924	0.023

Other Support Facilities Desired

Apart from the counseling service, the students were asked to describe what other support facilities they desired. After qualitative analysis of their desires, seven themes emerged as seen in Table 9.

Table 9. Other Support Facilities Desired by the Students

Support Facility	N %
Academic Support	251 (22.5)

Good Library
  Well Planned Academic Curriculum
  Better Teaching Aids
  Quality Teaching
  Computers/Access to Information
  Exchange Programme With Other Medical Schools
  Career Guidance
  Arrangements For Postings Missed
  Kinder Lecturer
  Lecturers Coming to Teach on Schedule
  Good Laboratory Equipment
  Smaller Student Groups	

Recreational/Sports Facilities	413 (36.9)

More Holidays
  Compulsory Recreational Course at Every Level of Study
  Basketball Courts
  Lawn Tennis -
  Internet Service-Cyber Café
  Functioning Swimming Pool
  Social Gatherings to Relieve Stress
  Well Equipped Gymnasium	

Utilities	373 (33.4)

Uninterrupted Power Supply/Generator
  Adequate Water Supply
  Proper Catering Service
  Proper Laundry Service
  Good Accommodation
  Direct Telephone – Access in Halls
  Shuttle Transport Between the University and the Teaching Hospital
  Better Intra Campus Transport Facilities
  Toilet in Every School Area – Neat/ Accessible
  Better Feeding Facility
  More Reading Rooms	

Financial Support	253 (22.6)

Student Loan System
  Financial Support
  Scholarships
  Vacation Jobs, Part Time Jobs
  Work In Laboratories/Kitchen Study	

Student-Faculty Information
  Feedback System Between Students And Lecturers
  Avenue to Lodge Complaints About Lecturers
  Suggestion Boxes For Students
  Students Well Educated on University Rules, Duties, Privileges.
  Avenue to Assess Performance of Faculty
	65 (5.8)

Support Facility	N %
Student Welfare Welfare Service For Students Special Support For Student Mothers Better Health Care System For Students	39 (3.9)
Other 'Seminars For the Girls on Dressing' 'Reduce Student Intake'	2 (0.2)

Discussion

Marked differences in the response rate to the questionnaire were noted across the different courses with the lowest response rates found among students studying medicine and dentistry. Several reasons may account for this observation. Students in the disciplines of Medicine and Dentistry who were on elective, rural and out-of-base postings could not be reached during the period of the study. Also, medical and dental students take clinical clerkships in several departments for varying lengths of time, making them less accessible when compared to the nursing and physiotherapy students who are fewer in number and do not receive academic instructions from so many different departments.

The age distribution in this study is characteristic of undergraduate samples where majority are below the age of 25 (Coletti et al., 2005). The representation of students in the study is in keeping with policy of the University to draw students from all over Nigeria. The University of Ibadan being the nation's premier University is under obligation to admit students from every state in the country. Naturally, the larger proportion of the students is drawn from the Southwestern part of the country where the university is located. The marked difference in the number of students from the Southeast and the South-south, when compared to the northern states, is indicative of the lower demand for university places among the people from the northern parts of the country.

Counseling Needs

In this study, academic counseling was the greatest counseling need of the students, followed by guidance in the areas of relationships, future career choices and financial issues. In the University of Toronto, the mental health professionals working in the student counseling service reported that 30%-40% of students coming for counseling had an academic need (Coletti et al., 2005). Students there also rated examination preparation (academics) as the most stressful occurrence requiring counseling, followed by career planning and finances. This pattern is similar to the counseling needs expressed by students in this study, except that in the Toronto study, students rated relationship problems after financial issues. On the other hand, at the Student Counseling Center at the University of Leeds, relationship problems were the biggest issue that counselors had to deal with. These relationship problems included those 'with family' in 15% of cases, 'with partner' in 8%, and 'with peers' in 8%. Academic counseling was needed in just 8% while mental health problems such as depression 9%, anxiety 8% were also reasons for seeking counseling

(Waller et al., 2005). Thus the pattern of demand among the students in Ibadan for counseling on academic issues and relationship problems does not differ much from what is found in the more developed areas of the world.

That about 5% of the students requested counseling on spiritual or religious issues is an interesting, if not surprising dimension in this environment. None of the university counseling services in the Western world that have been alluded to stated categorically that spiritual counseling was available (HUCS, 2002; Waller et al., 2005; Surtees et al., 2000). The demand for spiritual counseling in this environment however cannot be ignored. With nearly all the students claiming some form of religious affiliation, whether they described themselves as 'Pentecostal Christians', or as orthodox Christians or Muslims, it is obvious that they attach considerable importance to religion in their lives. This is a reflection of what is happening in the larger Nigerian society where participation in faith-based activities, particularly religious crusades, proselytization and overnight prayer vigils have become commonplace, affecting the lives and mental health of large numbers of people. Recent writings in Nigerian newspapers give credence to this trend. An example: 'Everyday people congregate in prayer houses, casting away and binding the devil. As early as 9am, they are already clapping, singing, dancing and chanting. In the night, they go for vigils, disturbing the neighborhood' (Igbokwe, 2005). A look at the students' requests under spiritual issues reveals that an important request was for counseling with regards to 'a balance between spiritual life and academics'. Although there is said to be an increasing awareness of the use of spiritual strategies in counseling in the developed world (Gubi, 2004), the students there do not seem to pay the same degree of attention to counseling in this area that the students in Nigeria do. Thus, this is an area of counseling that may require special emphasis in this environment.

Another counseling need mentioned by the participants in this study is 'difficulty with teachers', which was mentioned by nearly 5% of respondents. The hurt associated with this can be exemplified by some of the students' responses, expressed in their own words, as shown in Text Box 9: 'abuses by doctors on ward rounds as if there is something wrong with your head'. It is not clear if this pattern of abuse is peculiar to the health care professions (Wolf et al., 1992; Lebenthal et al., 1996; Kassebaum and Cutler, 1998) or cuts across all university areas (Coletti et al., 2005). However, what is apparent is an association between students experiencing abuse from their teacher and psychological distress in them (Omigbodun et al., 2004).

The request for counseling for utilities in this study is not unusual as students in a new environment such as a university would need guidance on obtaining accommodation. At the University of Edinburgh, where the student counseling service illustrates excellent collaborative work, one of the keys aspects of collaboration was in the area of providing university accommodation, including an accommodation service for students with disabilities (Jackson, 2002). However some of the requests for counseling by students in this study, as seen in Text Box 10, are unique requests to this developing country context. Inconsistent electricity supply and a lack of flowing tap water, insecurity and rising crime wave in the halls of residence are additional every day problems students in the environment have to contend with, in contrast to what obtains in other parts of the world where municipal services are taken for granted and better campus security is provided.

Though few, requests for counseling in the area of sexual harassment was made, this request must be taken seriously due to the potential adverse effects on affected students. In a graduating class of dental students in the USA (Wolf et al., 1992) sexual harassment was reported by a third of the students and it adversely affected different aspects of their lives. In this study, very few students requested for drug and alcohol counseling. The reasons for this are not clear because recent studies suggest that psychoactive substance use is a major problem among university undergraduates in Nigeria (Omigbodun and Babalola, 2004; Omokhodion and Gureje, 2003). It is possible that the students believe this problem is better handled elsewhere or could it be that students with drug use problems were in denial?

A common counseling area found in the developed country literature (Coletti et al., 2005), but which did not feature among the requests in this study is eating disorders. Adolescents with eating disorders are not yet reported in child and adolescent psychiatry samples in Nigeria (Omigbodun, 2004) and purposive surveys of this issue among university students are yet to be done to determine if it is a problem among them or not.

Association between Issues Triggering Counseling Requests and the Socio-Demographic Characteristics of the Respondents

The study of undergraduates in the University of Toronto did not find differences in counseling needs attributable to students' ages, year of study or course of study; only gender revealed differences (Coletti et al., 2005). In areas seen as stressful and requiring counseling such as examination preparation, course work deadlines, future career planning, relationships, finances and abuse or harassment, females rated higher. In this study however, several demographic factors showed a strong and independent relationship with the different requests for counseling.

Female students were more likely to request for academic counseling, male students for emotional counseling. As regards academic counseling it is not clear why females had an increased demand but from many of the descriptions (Text Box 1), it was evident that guidance in time management and being better organized for study was needed. The male students' higher demand for emotional counseling can be linked to the confidence building requests seen in Text Box 5. 'Losing confidence', 'how to enjoy life', 'motivation', 'when I'm angry I can't hide it', were some of the areas triggering counseling requests.

Age was associated with a request for financial counseling with students aged 31 years or more making a higher demand. Many more of these students were married with families. Some even had jobs, especially among the nurses, thereby having more income, more needs and a greater need for guidance on how to manage their finances.

Students who came from distant parts of the country to study were more likely to request for academic counseling. A close link is established between academic problems and psychological distress, and when students leave home, two key areas of support are removed: family and a familiar environment (Waller et al., 2005). In moving from one region to another in Nigeria, one meets with a completely new culture, different local language, manner of relating and all of these, added on to the stress of university life can contribute to the students' need for guidance and support with academic work.

Course of study also has fascinating connection with counseling requests in this cohort of students. The medical and dental students were more likely to request future career counseling than the nurses and physiotherapists. This is understandable because, in physiotherapy and nursing in this environment, opportunities for specialization are very limited and graduates go on to work and engage in further study as generalists. For the doctors and dentists however, things are different as they have greater opportunity for specialist training. Many move into residency training and they have to make important choices about what specialty to choose and where to undergo specialist training. Also counseling about family problems being in higher demand among the nursing and dental students may be linked to their having a family already. It is instructive to note that 47% of the nursing and 4% of the dental students were married, compared to only 1.2% of the medical and none of the physiotherapy students.

Levels of study also point to important details that need to be ironed out when developing counseling services. As seen in Table 3 and Figure 1, there are interesting trends in the pattern of counseling needs with increasing level of study. The greatest request for academic and emotional counseling is in the first year of study and this decreases progressively as the years go by, while it is the inverse when it comes to counseling needs in the area of future career plans. The complex interplay of academic and emotional needs (HUCS, 2002) are displayed here in the associated fall in these needs with rising level of study. The tremendous academic and emotional stress experienced by first year students was also illustrated in several other studies (Guthie et al., 1995; Lee and Graham, 2001). On the other hand as the time draws nearer for an end to undergraduate studies the crucial need for future career counseling builds up.

Counseling Needs and Psychological Distress

Four areas of counseling requests: academic issues, emotional problems, financial issues and utility problems are strongly and independently associated with evidence of psychological morbidity at a GHQ cut-off level of 3 or more. At even lower GHQ cut-offs of 2 or more the counseling requests are closely tied to evidence of psychological stress. This evidence further buttresses the finding of HUCS, (2002) that students presenting for counseling may be at risk for academic, emotional and financial problems and that there is a complex inter-relationship between these three factors. If the counseling facility is set up here, it becomes obvious that all students seeking counseling in these four areas should be assessed for mental health problems.

Need for Counseling Facilities

Almost half (47.4%) of the students indicated that they wanted a counseling service to be available for their use and three very important themes emerged from the qualitative analysis of responses of students who wanted a counseling service: a need to ventilate to obtain relief of tension, a need for information and guidance, and a need for information feedback to the authorities about their situation as students through the counseling service. The gender influences found on the emergent themes reveal some of the gender differences in needs for verbalization. That the female students wanted to ventilate and males wanted information is in keeping with research on gender differences in which females were found to be more emotionally sensitive than males and, except for anger, females were found to express their feelings more freely and intensely, using language, facial expressions and gestures, while men are found to be more interested in giving and receiving information (Berk, 1997; Pease and

Pease, 2002). In the University of Toronto study, counselors reported that women more readily confided about mental health issues and would seek professional help more often than the men (Coletti et al,, 2005).

On the other hand a small minority of 18% did not want a counseling service. Among the reasons they gave, three main themes are also evident and, on the face of it, appear legitimate. Money and utility problems may not be obviously amenable to counseling but what these students may have forgotten is what many of the students who wanted counseling felt: 'a problem shared is a problem half-solved'. Other themes include the need for lecturers to receive counseling themselves and the ability to take care of ones' self without counseling. The expressed need for lecturers to be counseled should be taken very seriously as many successful counseling programs have facilities not only to counsel lecturers but to train them to better understand the needs of students (Smith, 2002). That the students who reported that they could take care of themselves were more likely to be older suggests an increase in age being associated with greater independence.

Should Lecturers be the Counselors?

More students (39.4%) felt that lecturers should not be the counselors compared to those who felt that lecturers should provide counseling (34.8%). Of the students who had a positive attitude towards lecturers counseling, five themes emerged as the advantages of lecturers doing the counseling such as 'they have passed through similar stress before'. A closer look at these advantages revealed some limitations and additional things that require to be put into place for this to happen. These would include a need to select lecturers who are to serve as counselors based on their attitudes and personality, a need for training as counselors and limiting counseling by lecturers to the areas of academics and career choices. These themes also reveal hopes of the potential benefits that lecturers serving as counselors could bring, like improvement in their teaching and a positive enhancement of the lecturer-student relationship.

Reasons given by some students for not wanting their lecturers to counsel illuminates some of the critical areas where training and reorientation for faculty is urgently required. In an evaluation of a restructured personal tutor scheme at the University of Dundee Medical School (Malik, 2000), the students' readiness to discuss personal and academic problems with their tutor was found to be dependent upon the formation of a good relationship. It was this relationship that was most related to the perceived success of the scheme and the establishment of a good relationship was linked to the perceived approachability of the tutor.

At the University of Hertfordshire (HUCS, 2002), a course in student support and guidance is given once or twice a year for half a day over ten weeks and is open to any member of staff who has some responsibility for supporting students. Majority of the personnel that have attended the program have been academic staff, with all Faculties represented. At the end of the course, participants report a better understanding of students' issues, greater ability to identify when students need specialist help and a better understanding of the student support system service. Thus, when tackling the counseling needs of students, their teachers must not be left out. They must also be better equipped to deal with the demand such an involvement will place on them. The mental health of staff is affected by changes in curriculum, changes in their schedule of duties, and increased pressures on resources and time

(Stanley and Manthorpe, 2002), issues of contemporary relevance in the context of teachers taking on additional responsibility for counseling students.

Aspects of Counseling Requested by the Students

A description of features desired by the students in a counseling facility can be divided into 'the process desired' and 'the content desired'. A good atmosphere with a high premium placed on confidentiality while not losing sight of accessibility and affordability, with the availability of trained counselors are the key aspects of process desired. A broad content offering academic, emotional, spiritual and all the other counseling needs earlier stated in Table 1 is desirable. The service must also take into cognizance the ethnicity, cultural practices and belief systems of the potential users.

In designing a counseling service, it is important to build in collaboration and networking, as all these help to strengthen the core. This is clearly illustrated in the example of successful collaborative work of the University of Edinburgh, Student Counseling Service (HUCS, 2002). This service works with the University Health Service where most students are registered and which offers a weekly consultant psychiatric outpatient clinic. Also connected to the counseling service is the Disability Office, Students' Association, Nightline and University Accommodation Service.

Enlightenment campaigns and destigmatizing activities are also vital to the use of any counseling or mental health service. A survey of university counseling services in the UK (HUCS, 2002) reveal deeply ingrained enlightenment campaigns as it was found that over 80% of university counseling services offer training in mental health issues to staff and over 50% offer training to students, thereby raising awareness as to problems and consequences. Also at the University of Toronto Counseling Service advertisements were placed in the University newspaper to raise awareness, apart from the flyers and packages about counseling services handed to new students during the orientation week (Coletti et al., 2005).

An aspect not mentioned at all by participants in this study, as possible parts of a counseling service, are peer support programs whereby students are trained in basic counseling skills and thereafter they offer support to other students. This program was set up at the Oxford University in the UK to complement the University Counseling Service whereby peer supporters are the first stop for those with problems before they get too severe. An important component of this program is supervision of the supporters on a regular basis.

Willingness to Pay For Counseling Services

Most students were not willing to pay for a counseling service and those who were willing to pay were more likely to be nursing students. It is possible that the nurses had a better understanding of the need for counseling since courses in counseling are an important part of their curriculum and this informed their decision, but they were also more likely to have jobs and, hence, were more financially comfortable. As should be expected, students who reported difficult or desperate finances were not willing to pay for a counseling service. Most counseling services in the developed world offered counseling free to students as part of a package of university services, although if situations where a referral to a psychiatrist was necessary some payment was made, usually through health insurance. Presently in Nigeria, out-of-pocket payments are still the major method of healthcare financing and most would only proceed to hospital when situations get out of hand. Asking students from this kind of background to pay for counseling may be an exercise in futility.

Furthermore students with poor finances are already in a compromised situation and should be encouraged to seek help. Studies of university students in the UK revealed that depression occurred in a third of students who anticipated owing huge amounts of money compared to 8% among those who did not foresee such debts and anxiety occurred in 74% of those worrying about getting into debt compared to 45% of those not concerned about potential financial difficulties (Scott et al., 2001). One of the main sources of this financial problem was poor money management skills, such as careless budgeting and lack of self discipline. Also students believed that their financial problems affected their academic results. One of the recommendations made by the researchers was that money management lessons be introduced into the package of services rendered to students to help them become better managers of their finances.

Other Support Facilities Desired

A look at the additional support facilities desired reveals that what health care students in this part of world are asking for are basic process and content changes in their training and environment to make them better professionals. A good library, smaller student groups, uninterrupted electricity and water supply, feedback between lecturers and students, student intake to tally with facilities and free internet facilities.

Internet facilities that students in the developed world take for granted have to be paid for here on an hour-by-hour basis, often at exorbitant rates. The importance of integrating accessibility to the Internet into the package of regular services offered to students in this and other Nigerian universities cannot be overemphasized. Suggestions for counseling facilities include 'website for anonymous counseling', which would require unfettered access on the part of both the students and the counselors. Several universities in the developed world use the Internet as an integral part of their counseling services. At the University of Leeds, a student-friendly mental health advice website, which directs students to the right agencies for their problems and provides self help books that can be downloaded is in operation, and there is evidence from the number of hits that it is being greatly utilized by the students (Waller et al., 2005).

Conclusion and Recommendations

Among the students of this large university in Southwestern Nigeria, the major circumstances that they felt would make them seek guidance or counseling are academic problems, relationship/ courtship issues, future career choices, finances and emotional problems. These are also the major issues cited in similar surveys of students in the developed countries of the Western World. There is however a clearly articulated need for guidance on spiritual issues among students in this environment, which did not feature among their counterparts in the West.

The socio-demographic characteristics of the students in this university, notably age, gender, course of study, level (or year) of study, region of origin and self-reported financial situation, all had a discernible association with whether or not they perceived a need to seek counsel, as well as the aspects of their lives where they felt they could benefit from counseling. The level of study, in particular, demonstrated a clear dichotomy of trend, with counseling needs for academic and emotional problems declining with increasing number of years spent in the university while the need for career counseling followed an inverse trend. The self-perceived need for counseling among students showing evidence of psychological distress was significantly different from those of other students in four main areas: academic problems, emotional problems, financial problems and issues related to the provision of utilities.

The main features that students wanted in a counseling service were accessibility, affordability and the availability of trained counselors. Many students would prefer that their lecturers not do the counseling, while some would want access to an Internet-based counseling service.

It is obvious that there is an urgent need for the establishment of a formal counseling service in this university, and that it should be integrated into the existing package of services rendered to students. Requiring payment at the point of service may render it unaffordable, and consequently inaccessible to many of those who need the service most. It is preferable that professional counselors be engaged to provide the service but lecturers who receive special training and orientation in counseling techniques and students' needs could be engaged to counsel students, particularly on academic problems and future career choices.

References

Association for University and College Counselling AUCC (2001) *Annual Survey of Counselling in Further and Higher Education. 1999-2000*, Rugby: AUCC

Beck DL, Hackett MB, Srivastava R, Mckim E, Rockwell B (1997) Perceived level and sources of stress in university professional schools. *Journal of Nursing Education*, 36:180-186

Berk L. E (1997) *Child Development*. 4th Edition, Allyn and Bacon, Needham Heights, Massachusetts

British Association for Counselling and Psychotherapy (BACP) (2002) *Ethical Framework for Good Practice in Counselling and Psychotherapy*, Rugby: BACP

Caleb R, (2002) *Evaluation Study, Brunel University Counseling Service*. Brunel University, U.K.

Coletti S, Chow J, Hogarth S, Karim Z, Meiorin J (2005) *Assessing Perceptions of Mental Well-Being Among the University of Toronto Undergraduate Student Population: Recommendation For the Improvement of Counseling Services*. *http://www.cquest.utoronto.ca/env/env421h/healthut/mwb* (1st July 2005)

Dangerfield P (2001) Medical student debt in the United Kingdom. *Medical Education*, 35: 619-621

Egert S (1999) *Survey on Student Retention and Counseling*, Middlesex University, U.K.

Everly JS, Poff DW, Lamport N, Hamant C, Alvey G (1994) Perceived stressors and coping strategies of occupational therapy students. *American Journal of Occupational Therapy*, 48: 1022-1028

Firth J (1986) Levels and sources of stress in medical students. *British Medical Journal* 292: 1177-1180

Goldberg D, Williams P (1988) *A User Guide to the GHQ*. Windsor: NFER-Nelson

Gubi PM (2004) Surveying the extent of, and attitudes towards, the use of prayer as a spiritual intervention among British mainstream counselors. *British Journal of Guidance and Counseling,* 32; 4.

Gureje O, Obikoya B (1990) The GHQ as a screening tool in a primary care setting. *Social Psychiatry and Psychiatric Epidemiology* 25: 276-280

Guthie EA, Black D, Shaw CM, Hamilton J, Creed FH, Tomenson B (1995) Embarking upon a medical career: psychological morbidity in first year medical student. *Medical Education,* 29: 337-341

Heads of the University Counseling Services (HUCS) (2002) The impact of counseling services on Student Retention: *www.ad.rhul.ac.uk/counseling/retentionhtm* (29th June 2005)

Helmers KF, Danoff D, Steinert Y, Leyton M, Young SN (1997) Stress and depressed mood in medical students, law students, and graduate students at McGill University. *Academic Medicine* 72: 708-714

Henning, K., Ey, S., & Shaw, D. Perfectionism, the imposter phenomenon and psychological adjustment in medical, dental, nursing and pharmacy students. *Medical Education.* 1998; 32: 456-464

Humphris G, Blinkhorn A, Freeman R, Gorter R, Hoad-Reddick G, Murtomaa H, O'Sullivan R, Splieth C.(2002) Psychological stress in undergraduate dental students: baseline results from seven European dental schools. *European Journal of Dental Education,* 6(1): 22-29.

Igbokwe C (2005) Miracle and financial breakthrough. *The Sunday Punch,* Lagos, Nigeria. Thursday, July 28

Jackson S (2002) Successful Collaborative Work, Student Counseling Service, University of Edinburgh. (in) Heads of the University Counseling Services (HUCS) (2002) *The Impact of Counseling Services on Student Retention*: *www.ad.rhul.ac.uk/counseling/retentionhtm* (29th June, 2005)

Jones MC, Johnston DW (1997) Distress, stress and coping in first year student nurses. *Advances in Nursing,* 26: 475-82

Kassebaum DG, Cutler ER (1998) On the culture of student abuse in medical school. *Academic Medicine,* 73: 49-58

Lebenthal A, Kaiserman I, Lernan O (1996) Student abuse in medical school: a comparison of students' and faculty's perceptions. *Israeli Journal of Medical Science,* 32 (3-4): 229-238

Lee J, Graham AN (2001) Students' perception of medical school stress and their evaluation of a wellness elective. *Medical Education,* 35: 652-659

Malik S (2000) Students, tutors and relationships: the ingredients of a successful student support scheme. *Medical Education,* 34: 635-641

Morrison J (2001) More on medical student stress. *Medical Education,* 35: 617-618

Nolan R and Wilson V (1994) Gender and Depression in an Undergraduate Population. *Psychological Reports,* 1 75:1327-1330

Omigbodun OO (2004) Psychosocial issues in a child and adolescent psychiatric clinic population in Nigeria. *Social Psychiatry and Psychiatric Epidemiology,* 39 (8): 667-672

Omigbodun OO, Babalola O.(2004) Psychosocial dynamics of psychoactive substance misuse among Nigerian adolescents. *Annals of African Medicine,* 3(3): 111-115

Omigbodun O.O., Onibokun AC, Yusuf BO, Odukogbe AA, Omigbodun AO. (2004) Stressors and counseling needs of undergraduate nursing students in Ibadan, Nigeria. *Journal of Nursing Education*, 43(9): 412-415

Omokhodion FO, Gureje O. (2003) Psychosocial problems of clinical students in the University of Ibadan Medical School. *African Journal of Medicine and Medical Sciences*, 32(1): 55-58

Pease A, Pease B (2002) *Why Men Don't Listen And Women Can't Read Maps. How We Are Different And What To Do About It.* Orion Books Ltd, London

Radcliffe C, Lester H (2003) Perceived stress during undergraduate medical training: a qualitative study. *Medical Education*, 37:32-38

Rana R. (2000) *Counseling Students: a Psychodynamic Perspective*. Macmillan Press Ltd

Sanders AE, Lushington K. (2002) Effect of perceived stress on student performance in dental school. *Journal of Dental Education*, 66(1): 75-81

Scott, Lewis and Lea (eds) (2001) *Student Debt: The Causes and Consequences of Undergraduate Borrowing in the UK.* The Policy Press

Sheehan KH, Sheehan DV, White K, Leibowitz A, Baldwin DC Jr (1990) A pilot study of medical student 'abuse'. Students' perceptions of mistreatment and misconduct in medical school. *Journal of the American Medical Association*, 263: 533-537

Stanley N and Manthorpe J (eds) (2002) *Students' Mental Health Needs: Problems And Responses.* Jessica Kingsley Publishers

Supe AN (1998) A study of stress in medical students at Seth GS, Medical College. *Journal of Postgraduate Medicine*, 44: 1-6

Surtees P, Wainwright N, Pharoah P (2000) *Student Mental Health, Use of Services and Academic Attainment: A Report to the Review Committee of the University of Cambridge Counseling Service*

Timmins F, Kaliszer M. (2002) Aspects of nurse education programmes that frequently cause stress to nursing students—fact finding sample survey. *Nurse Education Today*, 22: 203-211

Waller R, Mahmood T, Gandi R, Delves S, Humphrys N, Smith D (2005) Student mental health: How can psychiatrists better support the work of university medical centres and university counseling services. *British Journal of Guidance and Counseling*, 33(1): 117-128

Wolf TM, Scurria PL, Bruno AB, Butler JA (1992) Perceived mistreatment of graduating dental students: a retrospective study. *Journal of Dental Education*, 56(5): 312-316.

In: Cancer Prevention Research Trends
Editors: Louis Braun and Maximilian Lange

ISBN: 978-1-60456-639-0
© 2008 Nova Science Publishers, Inc.

Chapter VII

Alternative Approaches to Cervical Cancer Prevention: Risk-Adapted Multimodal Laboratory Cervical Screening

Reinhard Bollmann[1], Alinda Dalma Varnai[1],
Agnes Bankfalvi[2,][*] and Magdolna Bollmann[1]
[1]Institute of Pathology, Bonn-Duisdorf, D-53124 Bonn, Germany;
[2]International Medical College (IMC), University of Münster, D-48147 Münster,
Germany.

Abstract

Cervical screening is acknowledged as currently the most effective approach for cervical cancer control. To date, there is extensive and strong evidence that cytology-based screening programs have been effective in reducing the incidence of and mortality from the disease in developed countries. However, conventional Papanicolaou (Pap) smears have inherent methodological shortcomings. New developments in cytology, such as liquid-based techniques and automated reading, seem to effectively overcome some of these limitations and have the potential to improve sensitivity and specificity of cytology both in diagnosis of and screening for cervical pre-cancer and cancer.

The recognition that cervical cancer is a consequence of an acquired infection with a few types of oncogenic human papillomaviruses (HPV) has led to novel opportunities for screening based on the use of HPV-tests. Current HPV testing systems are able to detect the presence of viral DNA in exfoliated cervical epithelial cells in close to 100% of invasive cervical cancer and up to 90% of its precursors. Thus, in terms of public health and also for practical purposes, all cervical cancer cases should be considered to be caused by HPV infection. A number of clinical studies have also demonstrated HPV testing to be more sensitive for the detection of clinically relevant pre-invasive cervical

---
[*] Correspondence concerning this article should be addressed to Dr Agnes Bánkfalvi, International Medical College (IMC), Gartenstrasse 21, D-48147 Münster, Germany. Tel: +49(0)251 210-86-39; Fax: +49(0)251 210-86-40; E-mail: bankfal@online.de.

disease than cytology alone and the combination of HPV tests and cytology may achieve a negative predictive value of >97% in detecting high grade intraepithelial neoplasia and cervical cancer.

However, in most women, cervical HPV infections remain asymptomatic and are transient, becoming undetectable in 1-2 years even by the most sensitive genetic tests. This is also true for high-risk HPV (HR-HPV) types. It is the long term persistence of certain HR-HPV genotypes that is strongly associated with cervical carcinogenesis in permissive cases. Therefore, discrimination between transient and persistent infections with a certain HPV genotype is essential for risk-adapted screening protocols, which can only be defined by genotyping of two consecutive probes.

Nevertheless, even the highly sensitive test combination of cytology and HR-HPV genotyping cannot predict the biological potential of prevalent cervical pre-cancers towards progression or regression. This can only be assessed by using an adequate biomarker of neoplastic transformation, e.g., DNA aneuploidy, in combination with morphological and HPV tests.

This review focuses on the clinical utility of conventional, ancillary and experimental methods for cervical screening and possible future directions for enhanced screening accuracy and prognostication using risk-adapted multimodal protocols.

Keywords: cervical screening, cytology, HPV-genotyping, DNA-cytometry

Current Epidemiological Status of Cervical Cancer – the European Union Perspective

Carcinoma of the cervix uteri is the second most common cancer in women worldwide with approximately 500 000 new cases diagnosed and 230 000 deaths each year. Almost 80% of new cases occur in the developing world where it is the leading cause of cancer-related death among women [1]. In the former European Union (EU), cervical cancer was estimated to comprise about 3% of cancers in women ranking eighth in importance and it was the tenth most common cause of cancer-related deaths in women in the year 1998 [2]. The recent expansion of the EU in May 2004 will certainly cause significant changes in cervical cancer rates, because there is a substantial excess in female mortality for the disease in most central and eastern European accession countries [3].

Cervical Screening – Past and Present

The objective of screening for cervical cancer is to reduce mortality and incidence of the disease. To date, there is extensive and strong evidence that this can be achieved by cytology-based screening programs as it was observed after the implementation of such regular population-based cervical screening in most developed countries in the 1960s. This has been mainly attributed to early detection and treatment of precancerous lesions. Where screening quality and coverage has been high, these efforts have reduced invasive cervical cancer by up to 90 percent [4,5]. Also in Germany, the age-standardized rates for cervical cancer incidence and mortality declined by 73% and 74% from 1960 to 1997 after the introduction of the statutory opportunistic cancer-screening program in the Western part of the country in 1971 [6]. Despite significant efforts in population-based screening that makes a free annual

Papanicolau (Pap) test available to all women 20 years of age and older covered by statutory health insurance (slightly above 90% of the adult female population) [7], the age-standardized annual incidence of 13.3 and mortality rate of 3.0 per 100000 women were among the highest in Europe in 2002 [8]. This can be partly explained by the generally poorer effectivity of an opportunistic screening program compared to an active invitation system [9].

In the meantime, accumulating data from organized screening programs indicate that the marked declines seen until the mid-1980s have been slowing and may even be increasing in certain countries [10]. This could reflect increased cancer detection by using new diagnostic techniques, such as human papillomavirus (HPV) testing and cervicography, or it might be the result of a cohort effect. Another factor with potential effect on incidence trends is the increase in rates of adenocarcinomas and adenosquamous carcinomas, which account for about 10% of all cervical cancers in Western populations [11]. These tumor types and especially their precursors are frequently missed by conventional Pap smears. These data suggest that the maximum effect of Pap smear-based screening could have been reached and further reduction in cervical cancer rates will require the introduction of new technologies and/or more efficient population screening strategies.

Cytology-Based Cervical Screening

Screening for cervical cancer and its precursors have been performed by the conventional Pap smear method over the last half-century [12] with well-published public health success and inherent methodological limitations. High-quality cytology is a highly specific screening test with estimates of 97% as the mean (range 86-100%). In contrast, sensitivity of a single smear may be between 30-87% (51% as the mean), although the sensitivity for high-grade disease alone is between 70% and 80% [13]. Put another way, although the specificity of the Pap test is generally very high, the sensitivity to detect cervical intraepithelial neoplasia (CIN) or invasive cancer is low with poor sample processing and interpretation errors being the major problems. Blood, mucus and drying artefacts contribute to the difficulty of identifying abnormal cells in the traditional Pap smear, and up to 10% of slides can prove unsuitable for interpretation, necessitating repeat visits and sampling [14]. Many of these problems can be overcome partially by improving methods of cell collection and presentation, but there remains a clear need to improve the traditional Pap test.

Newer technologies developed with the intention of improving cytological assessment include liquid-based cytology (LBC; ThinPrep, Autocyte), computerized re-screening (PAPNET), and algorithm-based computer re-screening (AutoPap). Several sub-optimal studies (split-sample or historical) have been performed to determine sensitivity, specificity and predictive values of these new methods; however lack of an adequate reference standard in most of the studies hampers proper assessment and comparison of test characteristics [15].

Nevertheless, the available evidence indicates that using liquid-based cytology, sensitivity is modestly higher for detecting any degree of cervical intraepithelial neoplasia (CIN), whereas specificity is modestly lower than with conventional Pap smears [13]. This supports the conclusion that liquid based cytology is an acceptable alternative to conventional cervical cytology smears, which is reflected by the Food and Drug Administration of the US (FDA) approval of two liquid-based Pap systems for routine use.

Even though several independent reviews on comparing liquid-based versus conventional cervical cytology came to the conclusion that there is no significant difference between the two methods [16,17], there are three major advantages of liquid based cytology over conventional Pap smears: i) numerous investigators agree that liquid based cytology markedly improves specimen adequacy [18-20], ii) the residual material can be used for ancillary testing (e.g., for HPV DNA), and iii) recent studies have shown an improvement in sensitivity and specificity for biopsy proven adenocarcinoma in situ (AIS) and adenocarcinoma [21,22].

Although LBC may improve the cytological identification of abnormal epithelial cells when they are present, the identification of such cells ultimately relies on the ability of the investigator to distinguish atypical cells from normal ones by conventional histochemical staining and microscopy, and to interpret their meaning for the patient. Thus, there is an inherent subjectivity in the traditional Pap-test. This led to the development of imaging systems that can enhance screening accuracy or even replace human investigators in the identification of aberrant cells [23]. Whether such systems should be used either in primary screening or to assist the cytologist in identifying abnormal cells is the subject of current debate.

Detection of HPV DNA as a Marker of Precursor Lesions

It is now well established that the vast majority of cervical carcinomas and its precursors worldwide are caused by persistent infections with certain high-risk types of human papillomaviruses (HR-HPV) [24-26]. Under optimal testing conditions, HR-HPV DNA can be identified in nearly all specimens of invasive cervical cancer (99.7%), in at least 70 % of CIN1, 80% of CIN2 and 96% of CIN3 precursor lesions. Using the Bethesda system nomenclature, HR-HPV DNA can be identified in some 50% of borderline cytology lesions (ASCUS), 80% of LSIL and 90-95% of HSIL and invasive cancer cases [27-28]. In terms of public health, these data indicate that the existence of HPV-negative cervical cancer cases is negligible and does not require any interventional targeting by screening.

However, epidemiologic studies have shown not only that women without HPV do not get cervical cancer but also that most women with HPV do not get cervical cancer. This is due to the fact that most HPV infections are transient in nature, especially in younger age groups, resulting either in no symptoms or minimal cellular changes, or low-grade intraepithelial lesions [29,30].

Research is ongoing to determine acceptable protocols for HPV testing for three main screening- or management-related purposes: 1) as primary screening in asymptomatic women with cytology results being negative for intraepithelial neoplasia or malignancy for estimating prevalence and distribution of HPV in the normal screening population and to define baseline HPV status in these women for diagnostic follow-up [31], 2) reflex HPV DNA testing for triage of women with initial equivocal and abnormal Pap smear (≥ ASCUS) [32], and 3) follow-up for treated cases for improved surveillance of residual disease and/or recurrence [33].

Primary screening studies have demonstrated HPV testing to be more sensitive than cytology alone, whereas the specificity of HPV-tests is age dependent. In the younger age groups, specificity is lower than for cytology and, in age groups of 35 years and older (also country-dependent); the specificity of tests is similar [32,34,35]. One of the strongest gains of the combination of HPV tests and cytology lies in the very high negative predictive value of >99% for detecting CIN3 or cancer [31]. Such a testing combination could potentially allow screening intervals to be increased; e.g. from the minimum of 3 years up to 5 years or longer, depending on the population and risk profile [36]. Furthermore, HPV DNA detection can successfully be performed on self-collected samples as well, which may be advantageous in specific patient groups [37]. Additionally, unlike the Pap smear, which can determine only whether abnormal cells are presently detected, molecular HPV testing has predictive value for lesions that may develop in the future [27,38]. HPV DNA testing also appears to represent a significant enhancement for detection of endocervical adenocarcinomas, which are otherwise difficult to detect and prevent [39]. One of the main drawbacks of this approach is the loss in specificity with respect to either test in isolation due to the excessive number of patients who would need to be referred for colposcopy [40]. Nevertheless, results from large investigational trials, including the ASC-US/Low-grade Squamous Intraepithelial Lesion (LSIL) Triage Study (ALTS), provide an abundance of data to justify the use of HPV testing for triaging ASC-US cases and as a follow-up test [41].

At present there are two HPV testing systems in widespread clinical use. Current hybrid capture technology (HC2 test) detects the presence of 13 types of oncogenic HPVs and 5 low-risk types using respective probe cocktails. Results are group-specific and do not allow distinction between different HPV genotypes. For clinical purposes, only the high-risk probe cocktail is used, with a reported sensitivity for detecting high- grade cervical intraepithelial neoplasias (CIN 2-3) between 84% and 100% [28,42,43].

However, because only women with long-lasting latent HPV infections, even with low levels of oncogenic types, are at high risk for developing HSIL [44], discrimination between transient and persistent infection with high-risk HPV types is essential for risk-adapted screening protocols. Furthermore, the persistence of at least one oncogenic HPV type is necessary for the emergency of pre-cancer [45], which can only be defined by genotyping of two consecutive probes because of the possibility of a new infection with another high risk type during the follow up period. Since the median duration of transient infection is 6 – 11 months [29,35], a second type (variant)- specific HPV test about 12 months after the first positive genotype-test should identify persistent type specific infections.

Genotyping can be performed by using different established PCR techniques (PGMY09/11-Amplicor LBA, GP5+/6+-EIA, SPF10-LIPA, PPF1/CP5-Sequencing) [46,47]. Amplified HPV DNA is identified by either microplate hybridization for detection of PCR amplicons (GP5+/6+-EIA) or a reverse hybridization line blot assay (PGMY09/11-LBA, SPF10-LIPA) that provides information on the specific type(s) detected [48,49].

It is significant that with the development of PCR-based HPV tests, new HPV genotypes are permanently detected with yet undefined-risk for cervical cancer. Furthermore, there is now evidence, that the different HR-HPVs can differ by an order of magnitude in risk for cervical cancer and during different morphological phases of the multi-step carcinogenesis, different HPV types have different oncogenic potential [50,51]. Therefore, the identification of prevalent HPV type may aid in the stratification of women who are at greatest risk for cervical cancer.

Although, simultaneous reporting of cytology and HPV results seems to be ideal, it is not always feasible, e.g. due to reimbursement issues in several countries. However, stringent cytomorphological criteria for minor HPV-associated cellular changes could help in pre-selecting high-risk patients with borderline smear abnormalities for subsequent molecular

HPV testing [20,52,53]. In our day-to-day diagnostic practice, the following non-classic features of HPV effect are assessed: i) *minor nuclear abnormalities* (mild hyperchromasia, mild nuclear variations and bi/multinucleation), ii) *disorders of keratinisation* (mild dyskeratosis and parakeratosis), iii) *measles cells and abortive koilocytes*, and iv) *degenerative changes* (macrocytes, cytoplasmic folding and keratohyalin-like granules). In a recent study we could show that all non-classic features were significantly associated with HPV in minimally abnormal cervical smears. Mild nuclear changes had 100% sensitivity and 100% negative predictive value for HPV infection [20]. Further, sensitivity and specificity of the combination of classical and non-classical HPV signs have nearly achieved 100% for PCR-based detection of HPV infection in women with squamous intraepithelial lesions (SIL) and high-grade intraepithelial lesions (HSIL), respectively [54,55]. Since >90% of HSIL is HPV infected, identification of even minor cytological changes suggestive of HPV infection could raise awareness of the screening cytologist more carefully to search for atypical cells. With complete lack of such minor abnormalities HPV infection and consequently the presence of HSIL is practically excluded and no further molecular HPV tests are needed.

Surrogate Biomarkers of Neoplastic Transformation

Theoretically, certain DNA, RNA or protein markers associated with neoplastic transformation of cervical epithelium subsequent to HPV infection could be applied in screening, diagnosis and prognosis. Because oncogenic HPVs are causative agents in cervical carcinogenesis and act via altering the cell cycle in infected epithelial cells, host genes interacting directly or indirectly with HPV oncoproteins have been extensively investigated in vitro [56,57]. The effect of the high-risk HPV early protein E7 on the function of the tumor suppressor pRB, which leads to over-expression of p16INK4A, a cyclin-dependent kinase inhibitor involved in cell cycle control has been investigated by several groups and a simple immunohistochemical assay has been developed for detecting p16 expression in both cell smears and tissue sections [58]. Diffuse, full thickness P16INK4A expression was found to discriminate low-grade from high-grade CIN and claimed to be a marker of high-risk HPV integration into DNA of infected squamous epithelial cells [59]. However, P16INK4A positivity in cervical glandular lesions was equivocal in different studies indicating limited utility of this biomarker in diagnosing suspicious glandular lesions, particularly in cytopathology [60].

Of markers of proliferative activity and differentiation, including Ki67, cell cycle regulators (Rb, p53, Cyclin A, E and D, p16, p21, p27, and telomerase), and cellular differentiation products (involucrin, CK13, CK14) combined quantitation of Ki67, Rb, CK13, and CK14 was found to predict progression risk of early CIN lesions [61].

From the above presentation of various putative molecular risk markers it is evident that no single marker reliably predicts the outcome of patients with abnormal cytology of any grade. A good candidate for a predictor of clinical outcome would be one that represents a wide range of significant genetic changes at early stages of carcinogenesis with a high positive and negative predictive value for abnormal and normal findings, respectively. Measurement of nuclear DNA content (DNA ploidy) is one approach that may fulfill these requirements. Normally, a non-dividing somatic cell contains 23 pairs or 46 chromosomes. This amount of DNA is called *diploid*. Just before cell division, the DNA is doubled and in mitosis, the 23 pairs of chromosomes are evenly distributed to two daughter cells. If no division follows the S-phase, the nucleus will then contain quadruples of DNA, making the cell *tetraploid*. Further doublings without cell division result in *polyploidy* that mean multiple copies of DNA in excess of diploidy. Polyploidisation often occurs in HPV infections, because the virus deranges the cell cycle. If the chromosomes are not uniformly distributed to the daughter cells or if parts of chromosomes become detached, the chromosomal segregation during mitosis is termed *unbalanced*. The unbalanced representation of chromosomes, i.e. gains or losses of chromosomal material, within nuclei is termed *aneuploidy*, which is a common feature in human cancers and pre-cancers [62].

Several lines of evidence indicate that aneuploidy is a cause rather than a consequence of malignant transformation and that it occurs early in carcinogenesis [63]. The development of genomic instability is an early and crucial event during HPV-associated cervical carcinogenesis, as well [64]. In line with others [65], we have recently reported that DNA ploidy measurement by image cytometry on cervical smears positive for HR-HPV help to detect women at high risk for developing high-grade cervical pre-cancer [66-68] This is supported by experimental results suggesting that increasingly deregulated expression of the E6-E7 oncogenes of HR-HPVs in epithelial stem cells first results in chromosomal instability and induces DNA aneuploidy followed either by subsequent integration of the HR-HPV genome into the affected cell clone [69] or alternative oncogene activation mechanisms [70]. Clinical studies support this concept in that cervical lesions with an aneuploid DNA profile are more likely to persist or progress than those with diploid or polyploid DNA content [71,72]. Thus, the assessment of DNA ploidy appears to have prognostic value in potentially malignant cervical lesions.

The method for measuring DNA ploidy uses automated image cytometry of nuclei from routinely processed cytology smears or separated nuclei from tissue samples, and needs little additional expertise over that currently available in most pathological laboratories.

Combination of Different Modalities

There is an increasingly large research literature on possible applications of new visual, microscopical and virological screening methods for prevention of cervical cancer [73]. Adding a second sensitive test to cytology, such as HR-HPV detection, yields a substantial increase in sensitivity and negative predictive value for high-grade CIN and cancer at the cost of concomitant decrease in specificity [35], which is of particular concern for large populations. A second test can be used sequentially as a triage method with the aim to restrict the number of screen-positives requiring referral. Among women with equivocal cytology results, HPV DNA testing is more accurate for detecting underlying CIN3 or cancer than repeat cytology. HPV DNA testing by virus group specific assays is not useful for triage of low-grade squamous intraepithelial lesions (LSIL in the Bethesda system) because of the very high HPV positivity [43]. Nevertheless, screening performance is largely influenced by population characteristics, especially the prevalence of underlying HPV infection. Therefore, all fundamental cervical screening statistics will vary greatly by region [73].

However, even the highly sensitive test combination of cytology and HR-HPV genotyping cannot assess the biological potential of prevalent cervical intraepithelial neoplasia towards progression or regression. An ideal test combination would indicate that an oncogenic HPV virus has already enhanced genetic instability and rendered cells susceptible to malignant transformation and consequent progression if left untreated. This can only be assessed by using adequate biomarkers in combination with morphological and/or HPV tests.

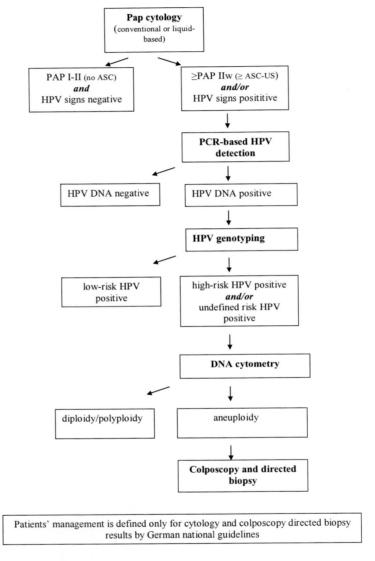

Figure 1. Risk-adapted, multimodal cervical screening program (the Bonn-scheme) using a combination of cytology and PCR-based HPV detection with adjuvant DNA-cytometry in the routine clinical setting. For the ideal case, the major steps include: 1) conventional Pap-test, or liquid-based cytology with special focus on assessing HPV-related cytomorphological changes (classic and non-classic HPV signs)(17), 2) cytology results of ≥PapIIw are managed by using reflex PCR-based HPV DNA testing, 3) in HPV DNA + cases, genotyping by sequencing, 4) in high-risk HPV+ cases, DNA cytometry for assessing gross chromosomal instability as progression marker (14), 5) only DNA aneuploid cases should be referred to immediate colposcopy and directed biopsy, 6) treatment is reserved for biopsy-confirmed ≥CIN3 cases 7) after ablation, Pap-smears are to be scheduled at 6-months with a repeated HPV DNA test.

Sporadic published results of such preliminary approaches are available only from experimental and/or study settings up to date [61,65,67,69-71]. Our institution is the first in Germany, which introduced a multimodal, risk-adapted cervical screening protocol using the combination of cytology, HPV genotyping and DNA image cytometry in a pure clinical setting including a routine screening population of about 30000 women from the Bonn-region in Western Germany. Since January 1999, all cervical samples from women sent to our institute by referral gynecologists from the region have been processed according to this screening profile (Figure1). Our preliminary results from the year 2002 based on samples from 123 women with ≥ASCUS cytology and concomitant cervical biopsy showed that the combination of all three test modalities resulted in up to 6.9% increase in positive predictive value (PPV) for moderate to high-grade cervical dysplasias and carcinomas (≥CIN2) compared to single tests or double combinations [74]. This combined approach had the additional benefit of being able to predict the possible outcome of histologically proven CIN1 lesions detected as false positives by single tests. Positivity for HR-HPV and DNA aneuploidy in a CIN1 lesion signalise a high risk for progression, whereas HR-HPV positivity with diploid DNA content indicate a probable benign course. Accordingly, our multimodal cervical screening protocol might permit identification of those women with low-grade squamous intraepithelial lesions (LSIL/CIN1) likely to progress at earlier and curable stage of disease and distinguish them from transient minor lesions caused by productive HPV infection. Our multimpodal screening and surveillance protocol may also help to individually predict the clinical outcome of cervical diseases post-surgery [75]. Using a combination of methods, although more expensive per screening, might be cost effective if the increased sensitivity permits lengthening of the screening interval in women at low risk for cancer development and progression [76,77]; and the ability to distinguish between low-worry and high-worry individuals could potentially reduce unnecessary invasive diagnostics and therapy with beneficial socio-economical impact.

Conclusion

To date, there are several good methods available for cervical screening. With appropriate screening programs and early diagnosis and treatment, cervical cancer may become a preventable public health issue in the foreseeable future. Based on good evidence, highly accurate screening for cervical cancer and high-grade intraepithelial neoplasias is now technically feasible. Given the abundant options for detecting its precursors, it is not a conceptual or technical challenge, but a matter of policy and financing which delays the elimination of this malignancy.

References

[1]   Parkin, DM; Bray, FI; Deves, SS. Cancer burden in the year 2000. The global picture. *Eur J Cancer* 2001;37: 4-66.

[2]   Ferlay, J; Bray, F; Sankila, R; Parkin, DM. *EUCAN: Cancer Incidence, Mortality and Prevalence in the European Union 1998.* version 5.0: IARC CancerBase No. 5. Lyon, IARC Press, 1999.

[3]   Levi F; Lucchini, F; Negri, E; La Vecchia, C. Trends in mortality from major cancers in the European Union, including acceding countries, in 2004. *Cancer* 2004; 101:2843-50.

[4]   Gustafsson, L; Ponten, J; Zack, M; Adami, HO. International incidence rates of invasive cervical cancer after introduction of cytological screening. *Cancer Causes Control* 1997; 8: 55-63.

[5]   Nieminen, P; Kallio, M; Hakama, M. The effect of mass-screening on incidence and mortality of squamous and adenocarcinoma of cervix uteri. *Obstet Gynecol* 1995; 85:1017-21.

[6]   Becker, N. Epidemiological aspects of cancer screening in Germany. *J Cancer Res Clin Oncol* 2003; 129:691-702.

[7]   Schenck, U; Karsa von, L. Cervical cancer screening in Germany. *Eur J Cancer* 2000; 36:2221-26.

[8]   Working group of population-based cancer registries in Germany: Krebs in Deutschland: Häufigkeiten und Trends. *www.rki.de/KREBS*; 2006.

[9]   Nieminen, P; Kallio, M; Anttila, A; Hakama, M. Organised vs spontaneous PAP-smear screening for cervical cancer: a case-control study. *Int J Cancer* 1999; 83:55-58.

[10]   Vizcaino, AP; Moreno, V; Bosch, FX; Munoz, N; Barros-Dios, XM; Parkin, DM. International trends in the incidence of cervical cancer: II Squamous cell carcinoma. *Int J Cancer* 2000;86:429-35.

[11]   Vizcaino, AP; Moreno, V; Bosch, FX; Munoz, N; Barros-Dios, XM; Parkin, DM. International trends in the incidence of cervical cancer: I Adenocarcinoma and adenosquamous carcionomas. *Int J Cancer* 1998; 75:536-45.

[12]   Papanicolau, GN. Survey on the actualities and potentialities of exfoliative cytology in cancer diagnosis. *Ann Int Med* 1949; 31:661-74.

[13]   Nanda, K; McCrory, DC; Myers, ER; Bastian, LA; Hasselblad, V; Hickey, JD; Matchar, DB. Accuracy of the Papanicolaou test in screening for and follow-up of cervical cytologic abnormalities: a systematic review. *Ann Intern Med* 2000;132:810-19.

[14]   Doorbar, J; & Cubie, H. Molecular basis for advances in cervical screening. *Mol Diagn* 2005;9:129-142.

[15]   Hartmann, KE; Nanda, K; Hall, S; Myers, E. Technologic advances for evaluation of cervical cytology: is newer better? *Obstet Gynecol Surv* 2001;56:765-74.

[16]   Davey, E; Barratt, A; Irwing, L; et al. Effect of study design and quality on unsatisfactory rates, cytology classifications, and accuracy in liquid-based versus conventional cervical cytology: a systematic review. *Lancet* 2006; 367: 122-32.

[17]   Obwegeser, J; Schneider, V. Thin-layer cervical cytology:a new meta-analysis. *Lancet* 2006; 367:88-89.

[18]   Diaz-Rosario, LA; Kabawat, SE. Performance of a fluid-based, thin-layer Papanicolaou smear method in the clinical setting of an independent laboratory and an outpatient screening population in New England. *Arch Pathol Lab Med* 1999;123:817-21.

[19]   Saslow, D; Runowicz, CD; Solomon, D; et al. American Cancer Society Guideline for the early detection of cervical neoplasia and cancer. *CA Cancer J Clin* 2002;52:342-62.

[20]   Bollmann, M; Bánkfalvi, A; Trosic, A; Speich, N; Schmitt, C; Bollmann, R. Can we detect cervical human papillomavirus (HPV)-infection by cytomorphology alone? Diagnostic value of non-classic cytological signs of HPV effect in minimally abnormal Pap tests. *Cytopathology* 2005;16: 13-21.

[21]   Bai, H; Sung, CJ; Steinhoff, MM. ThinPrep Pap test promotes detection of glandular lesions of the endocervix. *Diagn Cytopathol* 2000;23:19-22.

[22]   Ashfaq, R; Gibbons, D; Vela, C; Saboorian, MH; Iliya, F. ThinPrep Pap Test. Accuracy for glandular disease. *Acta Cytol* 1999;43:81-85.

[23]   Wilbur, DC. Cervical cytology automation: an update for 2003. The end of the question nears? *Clin Lab Med* 2003; 23:755-74.

[24]   Schiffman, MH; Bauer, HM; Hoover, RN; et al. Epidemiologic evidence showing that human papillomavirus infection causes most cervical intraepithelial neoplasia. *J Natl Cancer Inst* 1993;85:958-64.

[25]   Bosch, FX; Manos, MM; Munoz, N; et al. Prevalence of human papillomavirus in cervical cancer: a worldwide perspective. International biological study on cervical cancer (IBSCC) Study Group. *J Natl Cancer Inst* 1995;87:796-802.

[26]   Walboomers, JMM; Jacobs, MV; Manos, MM; et al. Human papillomavirus is a necessary cause of invasive cervical cancer worldwide. *J Pathol* 1999;189:1–3.

[27]   Nobbenhuis, M; Walboomers, JM; Helmerhorst, TJ; et al. Relation of human papillomavirus status to cervical lesions and consequences for cervical-cancer screening: a prospective study. *Lancet* 1999; 354:20–25.

[28]   Clavel, C; Masure, M; Bory, JP; et al. Human papillomavirus testing in primary screening for the detection of high-grade cervical lesions: a study of 7932 women. *Br J Cancer* 2001;84:1616-23.

[29]   Ho, GY; Bierman, R; Beardsley, L; Chang, CJ; Burk, RD. Natural history of cervicovaginal papillomavirus infection in young women. *N Engl J Med* 1998; 338:423-8.

[30]   Moscicki, AB; Shiboski, S; Hills, NK; et al. Regression of low-grade squamous intra-epithelial lesions in young women. *Lancet* 2004; 364:1678-83.

[31]   Sherman, ME; Lörincz, AT; Scott, DR; Baseline cytology, human papillomavirus testing and risk for cervical neoplasia: a 10-year cohort analysis. *J Natl Cancer Inst* 2003; 95:46-52.

[32]   Schiffman, M; Herrero, R; Hildesheim, A; et al. HPV DNA testing in cervical cancer screening: results from women in a high-risk province of Costa Rica. *JAMA* 2000;283:87-93.

[33]   Wright, TC; Schiffman, M; Solomon, D; et al. Interim guidance for the use of human papillomavirus DNA testing as an adjunct to cervical cytology screening. *Obstet Gynecol* 2004; 103:304-9.

[34]   Schneider, A; Hoyer, H; Lotz, B; et al. Screening for high-grade cervical intra-epithelial neoplasia and cancer by testing for high-risk HPV, routine cytology or colposcopy. *Int J Cancer* 2000; 89:529-34.

[35]   Cuzick, J; Szarewski, A; Cubie, H; et al. Management of women who test positive for high-risk types of human papillomavirus: the HART study. *Lancet* 2003; 362:1871-6.

[36]   Advisory Committee on Cancer Prevention. Recommendations on cancer screening in the European Union. *Eur J Cancer* 2000; 36:1473-78.

[37]   Dannecker, C; Siebert, U; Thaler, CJ; Kiermeir, D; Hepp, H; Hillemanns, P. Primary cervical cancer screening by self-sampling of human papillomavirus DNA in internal medicine outpatient clinics. *Ann Oncol* 2004;15:863-9.

[38]   Schlecht, NF; Platt, RW; Duarte-Franco, E; et al. Human papillomavirus infection and time to progression and regression of cervical intraepithelial neoplasia. *J Natl Cancer Inst* 2003; 95:1336-43.

[39]   Davey D; & Zarbo, RJ. Human papillomavirus testing – Are you ready for a new era in cervical cancer screening? *Arch Pathol Lab Med* 2003; 127:927-29.

[40]   Franco, EL.Chapter 13: Primary screening of cervical cancer with human papillomavirus tests. *J Natl Cancer Inst Monogr* 2003; 31:89-96.

[41]   Schiffman, M; Solomon, D. Findings to date from the ASCUS-LSIL Triage study (ALTS). *Arch Pathol Lab Med* 2003; 127:946-49.

[42]   Wright, TC; Denn, L; Kuhn, L; Pollack, A; Lorincz, A. HPV DNA testing of self-collected vaginal samples compared with cytologic screening to detect cervical cancer. *JAMA* 2000; 283: 81-86.

[43]   Arbyn, M; Buntinx, F; Van Ranst, M; et al. Virologic versus cytologic trial of women with equivocal Pap smears: a metaanalysis of the accuracy to detect high-grade intraepithelial neoplasia. *J Natl Cancer Inst* 2004; 96:280-93.

[44]   Ho, GY; Burk, RD; Klein, S; et al. Persistent genital human papillomavirus infection as a risk factor for persistent cervical dysplasia. *J Natl Cancer Inst* 1995; 87:1365-71.

[45]   Kjaer, SK; van den Brule, AJ; Paul, G; et al: Type specific persistence of high risk human papillomavirus (HPV) as indicator of high grade cervical squamous intraepithelial lesions in young women: population based prospective follow up study. *BMJ* 2002; 325:1-7.

[46]   Coutlee, F; Gravitt, P; Kornegay, J; et al. Use of PGMY primers in L1 consensus PCR improves detection of human papillomavirus DNA in genital samples. *J Clin Microbiol* 2002; 40:902-7.

[47]   Poljak, M; Marin, IJ; Seme, K; Vince, A. Hybrid Capture II HPV Test detects at least 15 human papillomavirus genotypes not included in its current high-risk probe cocktail. *J Clin Virol* 2002; 25 Suppl 3: S89-97.

[48]   Kay, P; Meehan, K; Williamson, AL. The use of nested polymerase chain reaction and restriction fragment length polymorphism for the detection and typing of mucosal human papillomaviruses in samples containing low copy numbers of viral DNA. *J Virol Methods* 2002; 105:159-70.

[49] Perrons, C; Kleter, B; Jelley, R; Jalal, H; Quint, W; Tedder, R. Detection and genotyping of human papillomavirus DNA by SPF10 and MY09/11 primers in cervical cells taken from women attending a colposcopy clinic. *J Med Virol* 2002; 67:246-52.

[50] Munoz, N; Bosch, FX; de Sanjose, S; et al. Epidemiologic classification of human papillomavirus types associated with cervical cancer. *N Engl J Med* 2003; 348:518-27.

[51] Bolkmans, NW; Bleeker, MC; Berkhof, J; Voohosrt, FJ; Snijders, PJ; Meijer, CP. Prevalence of types 16 and 33 is increased in high-risk human papillomavirus positive women with cervical intraepithelial neoplasia grade 2 or worse. *Int J Cancer* 2005; 117:177-181.

[52] Schneider, A; Meinhardt, G; de Villiers, EM; Gissmann, L. Sensitivity of the cytologic diagnosis of cervical condyloma in comparison with HPV DNA hybridization studies. *Diagn Cytopathol* 1987; 3:250-5.

[53] Checchini, S; Confortini, M; Bonardi, M;et al. "Nonclassic" cytologic signs of cervical condyloma. *Acta Cytol* 1990; 6:781-4.

[54] Bollmann, R; Mehes, G; Torka, R; Speich, N; Schmitt, C; Bollmann, M. Human Papillomavirus Typing and DNA Ploidy Determination of Squamous Intraepithelial Lesions in Liquid-Based Cytologic Samples. *Cancer Cytopathol* 2003; 99:57-62.

[55] Speich, N; Schmitt, C; Bollmann, R; Bollmann, M. Human papillomavirus (HPV) study of 2916 cytological samples by PCR and DNA sequencing: genotype spectrum of patients from the west German area. *J Med Microbiol* 2004; 53:1-4.

[56] Alazawi, W; Pett, M; Arch, B; Scott, L; Freeman, T; Stanley, MA; Coleman, N. Changes in cervical keratinocyte gene expression associated with integration of human papillomavirus 16. *Cancer Res* 2002; 62:6959-65.

[57] Al Moustafa, AE; Foulkes, WD; Wong, et al. Cyclin D1 is essential for neoplastic transformation induced by both E6/E7 and E6/E7/ErbB-2 cooperation in normal cells. *Oncogene* 2004; 23:5252-6.

[58] Klaes, R; Friedrich, T; Spitkovsky, D; et al. Overexpression of P16INK4a as specific marker for dysplastic and neoplastic epithelial cells of the cervix uteri. *Int J Cancer* 2001; 92: 276-84.

[59] Hu, L; Guo, M; He, Z; Thornton, J; McDaniel, LS; Hughson, MD. Human papillomavirus genotyping and p16(INK4a) expression in cervical intraepithelial neoplasia of adolescents. *Mod Pathol* 2005; 18:267-73.

[60] Murphy, N; Heffron, CC; King, B; et al. P16(INK4A) positivity in benign, premalignant and malignant cervical glandular lesions: a potential diagnostic problem *Virchows Arch* 2004;445:610-15.

[61] Kruse, AJ; Skaland, I; Janssen, EA; et al. Quantitative molecular parameters to identify low-risk and high-risk early CIN lesions: role of markers of proliferative activity and differentiation and Rb availability. *Int J Gynecol Pathol* 2004; 23:100-9.

[62] Sen, S. Aneuploidy and cancer. *Curr Opin Oncol* 2000; 12:82-8.

[63] Duesberg, P; & Li, R. Multistep carcinogenesis. A chain reaction of aneuploidizations. *Cell Cycle* 2003; 2:202-210.

[64] zur Hausen H. Papillomavirus causing cancer: evasion from host cell control in early events in carcinogenesis. *J Natl Cancer Inst* 2000; 92:690-698.

[65] Lorenzato, M; Bory, JP; Cucherousset, J; et al. Usefulness of DNA ploidy measurement on liquid-based smears showing conflicting results between cytology and high-risk human papillomavirus typing. *Am J Clin Pathol* 2002; 118:708-13.

[66] Bollmann, R; Bollmann, M; Henson, DE; Bodo; M. DNA cytometry confirms the utility of the Bethesda system for the classification of Papanicolaou smears. *Cancer Cytopathol* 2001 93:222-8.

[67] Bollmann, R; Mehes, G; Torka, R; Speich, N; Schmitt, C; Bollmann M. Determination of features indicating progression in atypical squamous cells with undetermined significance: human papillomavirus typing and DNA ploidy analysis from liquid-based cytologic samples. *Cancer* 2003; 99:113-17.

[68] Bollmann, R; Mehes, G; Speich, N; Schmitt, C; Bollmann, M. Aberrant, highly hyperdiploid cells in human papillomavirus positive, abnormal cytologic samples are associated with progressive lesions of the uterine cervix. *Cancer Cytopathol* 2005; 105:96-100.

[69] Melsheimer, P; Vinokurova, S; Wentzensen, N; Bastert, G; von Knebel-Doeberitz, M. DNA aneuploidy and integration of human papillomavirus type 16 e6/e7 oncogenes in intraepithelial neoplasia and invasive squamous cell carcinoma of the cervix uteri. *Clin Cancer Res* 2004; 10:3059-63.

[70] Sathish, N; Abraham, P; Peedicayil, A; Sridharan, G; John, S; Chandy G. Human papillomavirus 16 E6/E7 transcript and E2 gene status in patients with cervical neoplasia. *Mol Diagn* 2004; 8:57-64.

[71] Bibbo, M; Dytch, HE; Alenghat, E; Bartels, PH; Wied, GL. DNA ploidy profiles as prognostic indicators in CIN lesions. *Am J Clin Pathol* 1989; 92:261-65.

[72] Bocking, A; Nguyen, VQ. Diagnostic and prognostic use of DNA image cytometry in cervical squamous intraepithelial lesions and invasive carcinoma. *Cancer Cytopathol* 2004;102:41-54.

[73] Ferreccio, C; Bratti, MC; Sherman, ME; et al. A comparison of single and combined visual, cytologic, and virologic tests as screening strategies in a region at high risk of cervical cancer. *Cancer Epidemiol Biomarkers Prev* 2003; 12:815-23.

[74] Bollmann, R; Bankfalvi, A; Griefingholt, H; et al. Validity of combined cytology and human papillomavirus (HPV) genotyping with adjuvant DNA-cytometry in routine cervical screening: results from 31031 women from the Bonn-region in West Germany. *Oncol Report* 2005; 13:915-922

[75] Bollmann, M; Varnai, AD; Griefingholt, H; et al. Predicting treatment outcome in cervical diseases using liquid-based cytology, dynamic HPV genotyping and DNA cytometry. *Anticancer Res* 2006; 26:1439-46.

[76] Maxwell, GL; Carlson, JW; Ochoa, M; Krivak, T; Rose, GS; Myers, ER. Costs and effectiveness of alternative strategies for cervical cancer screening in military beneficiaries. *Obstet Gynecol* 2002; 100: 740-748

[77] Goldie, SJ; Kim, JJ; Wright, TC. Cost effectiveness of human papillomavirus DNA testing for cervical cancer screening in women aged 30 years or more. *Obstet Gynecol* 2004; 103:619-631

In: Cancer Prevention Research Trends
Editors: Louis Braun and Maximilian Lange

ISBN: 978-1-60456-639-0
© 2008 Nova Science Publishers, Inc.

Chapter VIII

Can a Home-Visit Invitation Increase Pap Smear Screening in Samliem, Khon Kaen, Thailand?

W. Chalapati and B. Chumworathayi*

Department of Obstetrics and Gynecology, Faculty of Medicine, Khon Kaen University,
Khon Kaen, 40002, Thailand. Tel; 66-4336-3030, Fax; 66-4334-8395

Abstract

Objective

To assess the efficiency of a home-visit invitation aimed to increase uptake of cervical cancer screening in women between 35 and 60 years of age.

Method

Since May, 2006, we conducted a quasi-randomized trial to determine if an in-home education and invitation intervention would increase uptake of cervical cancer screening. We randomly recruited 304 women from the Samliem inner-city community, Khon Kaen, Northeast Thailand, and assigned participants to either the intervention or control zone. Baseline screening coverage interviews were then done: 58 of 158 women in the intervention zone and 46 of 146 in the control zone were excluded from the study because of having had a Pap smear within 5 years, but these were included in the final analysis. First, 100 women in the intervention group were visited in their homes by one of the researchers, who provided culturally-sensitive health education that emphasized the need for screening. Four months later, post-intervention, screening-coverage

---

* Correspondence: Asst. Prof. Dr. Bandit Chumworathayi, MD. Department of Obstetrics and Gynecology, Faculty of Medicine, Khon Kaen University, Khon Kaen, Thailand, 40002. Tel; 66-4336-3030, Fax; 66-4334-8395, E-mail; chumworathayi@thai.com

interviews were again performed in both groups, in combination with the same health education for 100 women in the control group for a comparison.

Results

There was no difference in the baseline Pap smear screening-coverage rate in the intervention *vs.* control zones (36.7 *vs.* 31.5%, p=0.339). One hundred women in the intervention group completed the intervention interviews and after four months, 100 women in the intervention group and 100 in the control group also completed the post-intervention interviews. The increased screening-coverage rate in the intervention zone was similar to that of the control zone (43.6 *vs.* 34.9%, p=0.119); however, there was a borderline significant increase in the intervention zone compared with baseline (36.7 to 43.6%, p=0.070).

Conclusion

Home visit education and invitation intervention produced a borderline significant effect on increasing Pap smear coverage within 4 months of study period.

Keywords: Pap smear, cervical cancer; screening coverage

Introduction

Cervical cancer is the third most common cancer worldwide, with at least 400,000 new cases identified throughout the world each year. Eighty percent of these cases occur in developing countries where some 200,000 die as a result of cervical cancer every year [1].

Cervical cancer is potentially one of the most preventable cancers, unlike many other cancers, because it is easily detectable and has a prolonged pre-malignant phase [2]. The Papanicolaou, or Pap smear, is a screening test used worldwide, primarily for the detection of precancerous changes within the cervix (i.e., abnormalities in the cells of the cervix known as dysplasia) [3].

The WHO has calculated the level of protection women gain as a population by regular screening and the number of tests they will need in a lifetime. An annual screening smear provides a 93.5% reduction in the incidence of cervical cancer and screening every 5 years provides an 85% reduction [4]. Due to limited resources, Thailand has a screening policy of every 5 years for women between 35 and 65 years of age.

There are several reasons why women developing invasive cervical cancer fail to have cancer detected at a pre-invasive stage by screening [7,8]: (1) primarily because they have never been screened at all [9-14]; and, (2) secondarily a lack of knowledge or awareness. The latter could be improved by health education and direct invitations to undergo a Pap smear during regular home visits by community-based healthcare professionals.

In Thailand, cervical cancer is the most common female cancer, killing ~5,000 annually and increasing. A multi-province survey by the Thai National Cancer Institute found that coverage of the previous cervical cancer screening program (i.e., the opportunistic Pap smear) was only 5% [5] compared with the WHO target of 80%. [6]

A systematic review published in 2005 in The Cochrane Database shows that invitations are an effective method of increasing uptake of cervical cancer screening. However, the majority of studies reviewed were from developed countries; thus, their relevance to developing countries is unclear [15].

A study was conducted with the aim of determining coverage in a defined population in Thakaserm sub-district in Nampong district, a rural area of Khon Kaen Northeast, Thailand. All women 20 and over were asked to complete a questionnaire and a total of 1,199 responded, of whom 66.9% reported having had a Pap smear test at least once, while 33.1% had never had one [16]. Coverage of Pap smear screening every 5 years among Khon Kaen inner-city women is thought to be even lower than this.

To reduce the incidence and mortality of cervical cancer among Thai women, we designed this study to assess the efficiency of a home visit invitation intervention to increase uptake of cervical cancer screening among women between 35and 60 years of age to the WHO recommendation.

Materials and method

Samliem community is a large community located near Khon Kaen University campus; therefore, 1 to 1.5 km (10-15 min on foot) from Srinagarind (university) Hospital and not more than 500 m from a community health station where women can get a Pap smear.

We designed this study as a quasi-randomized trial to answer the question, "Can home visit invitation increase uptake of Pap smear testing?" We subdivided the community into intervention or control zones in May, 2006. By a random walking survey, we randomly selected 304 women between 35 and 60 years of age within these 2 zones for interviews.

This design was used to decrease bias and data contamination because of the short distance between respondents' homes. Women, who had undergone a Pap smear within five years, had previously had an abnormal Pap smear, had no cervix or were terminally ill, were excluded.

Sample size was calculated from our pilot study, which indicated that Pap smear coverage in this community was 30%, and we expected to see an increase to 50% four months after intervention. With a power of 80%, $Z_\beta=0.84$ and $Z_\alpha=1.96$, we needed at least 93 women in each zone. We were, however, able to provide intervention and interviews for 100 eligible women in each study group. We, thus, collected data on Pap smear coverage within 5 years in each group by asking all of the selected women until we reached 100 eligible women (i.e., those not excluded by any of the above criteria) in each zone for the intervention and control groups. Finally, 158 and 146 women comprised the intervention and control groups, respectively (Figure 1).

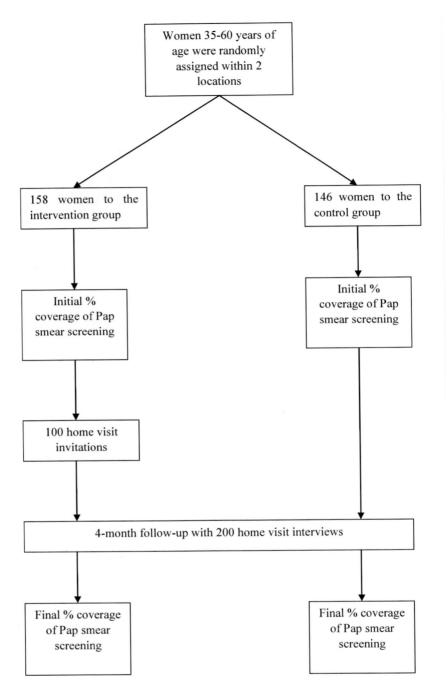

Figure 1. Participant flow chart.

One-hundred women randomly selected in the first zone were assigned to an intervention group (which would get a home-visit invitation) while 100 women in the second location were assigned to the control group. We first gathered baseline information on both groups by Family Practitioner Nurses based at the Samliem Health Station, through interviews of all 200 women (i.e., name, date of birth, address, marital status, parity, education, career and monthly income) during the first home visit. No intervention was given during the first home visit. Then within the month of May, 2006, all of the women in the intervention group had the study explained to them and they then provided informed consent as per the requirements of our institutional ethics review board.

Participants were visited at home and shown the leaflet then given the short questionnaire. After the interview, each woman was left with a fact sheet for further reading. All of the interviews and invitations to have an annual Pap smear check-up were done by one of the authors (WC) and lasted between 45 min and 1 hr. The outcomes of the intervention were evaluated during a third home visit interview four months after the first home visit invitations by the same author. By this time (September, 2006), all of the women in the control group would have had the same intervention as the first group.

Results

Samliem community has a total population of 12,942; of whom 6,694 are women and of these 1,905 are between 35 and 60 years of age. The intervention zone (Moo 14) has a total female population of 3,842 with 789 between 35 and 60; while the control zone (Moo 16) has a total female population of 9,130 with 1,796 between 35 and 60. Of the 304 women selected at random from the two zones of this inner-city community, we successfully recruited 200 (65.8%); that is, they had none of the exclusion criteria.

We excluded 104 (34.2%) because their previous Pap smear was done within the past 5 years. The coverage of Pap smear among women 35-60 years-old--*according to the Thai national cervical cancer screening program (every 5 years)*--was 34.2%. No other exclusion criteria were found.

Our randomization successfully yielded two comparable study groups. There was no significant or practical difference between these two groups in the distribution of subjects by age, marital status, parities, educational level, employment status or income (Table 1). Both groups were similar in their baseline cervical cancer screening practices (Table 2); that is, 86% of the participants in the intervention group had received a Pap smear >5 years prior to the baseline interview *vs.* 78% in the control group (p=0.136). One hundred women (100%) in the intervention group participated in the intervention interviews (at the beginning) and one hundred women (100%) in the control group also participated in the post-intervention interviews (at the end). This means that all 200 women in both groups (100%) received a home visit invitation and health educational session.

Among the 200 women not obtaining recommended screening exams at baseline, there were substantial increases in Pap smear screening among both the intervention and control groups (Table 3). These improvements were similar between groups (11 *vs.* 5, p=0.136). The reasons why 89 and 95 of the women in the intervention and control group did not get a Pap smear after 4 months were similar: (1) no occasion, (2) no symptoms, (3) shame, and, (4) fear of pain.

We asked participants, What strategies would encourage them to get a Pap smear? They answered similarly: (1) sending out a mobile unit, (2) giving them an appointment, and (3) using supporting activities (i.e., special holidays, mass screening with friends, or even a legal requirement). However, some participants said that no external organized incentive would help because getting a smear would always depend upon circumstances. These proposed strategies were not significantly different between groups except that the intervention group proposed the mobile unit less frequently than the control group (i.e., 27% *vs.* 53%, p<0.001).

We were interested in, "Why 5 women in the control group went for Pap smears?" The replies include: fear of cancer (3), due to a health volunteer's advice (1), and because an annual check-up was provided at work (1). The first three affirmed that they did not know the results of such investigations from other women in the intervention zone. Therefore, we are reasonably confident that there was no contamination between both groups.

The final analysis--*based on the whole sample, including those who were previously excluded*--assumed that screening coverages were similar to baseline practices. This comparison found slight increases in Pap test screening rates among both groups in the intervention zone (36.7 to 43.6%, p=0.070) and in the control zone (31.5 to 34.9%, p=0.374) (Table 4). Women in the intervention zone had a somewhat greater increase in Pap smear coverage rates from baseline, but the observed difference was of borderline statistical significance (36.7 to 43.6%, p=0.070). There was no significant difference between zones in either the initial (36.7 *vs.* 31.5%, p=0.339) or final coverage rates (43.6 *vs.* 34.9%, p=0.119). In conclusion, the intervention and control zones improved their Pap smear screening coverage rate without significant levels between the initial and final surveys.

Table 1. Comparison of demographic data between the two groups

Characteristics	Intervention group N=100 Mean or number	Control group N=100 Mean or number	P-value*
Age (mean in years)	46.97	47.37	0.719
Marital status			
Single	87	86	1.000
Married	13	14	
Parities (mean)	2.09	2.50	0.345
Educational level			
Primary school	54	53	0.863
Secondary school	25	23	
Bacheler degree or higher	21	24	
Employment status			
Household worker	45	49	0.790
Private business employee	5	5	
Private business owner	32	33	
Government officer	18	13	
Income/month			
<5,000 THB	32	37	0.662
5,001-10,000 THB	27	30	
10,001-15,000 THB	21	13	
15,001-20,000 THB	11	11	
20,001-25,001 THB	9	9	

*The χ^2 and Fisher's exact test was used for the continuous and categorical data, respectively.

Table 2. Baseline practices vis-à-vis annual Pap smear screening

Practices	Intervention group N %	Control group N %	P-value*
1. Previous pelvic exam			
▪ Yes	86	78	0.136
▪ No	13	22	
2. Reasons for exam			
▪ Check-up	27	19	0.240
▪ Leukorrhea	13	15	0.684
▪ Itching	10	16	0.293
▪ Bleeding	5	4	0.999
▪ Pain	14	17	0.558
▪ Dysmenorrhea	7	4	0.535
▪ Mass	2	1	0.999
▪ Infertility	1	0	0.999
▪ Postpartum	46	52	0.479
▪ Dysuria	3	3	0.999
▪ Others	4	2	0.683
3. Reasons for non-exam			
▪ No symptoms	10	15	0.392
▪ Shame	5	14	0.054
▪ Fear of pain	5	2	0.445
▪ Other	6	0	0.029
4. Cervical cancer awareness			
▪ Yes	84	92	0.128
▪ No	16	8	
5. Previous Pap smear			
▪ Yes	70	75	0.526
▪ No	30	25	
6. Time since last Pap smear			
▪ 5 years	37	36	0.509
▪ >5 years	33	40	
▪ Never had	30	24	
7. Reasons for never having Pap smear			
▪ No symptoms	21	19	0.860
▪ Shame	12	13	1.000
▪ Fear of pain	11	3	0.052
▪ Other	8	3	0.215

*The χ^2 and Fisher's exact test was used for the continuous and categorical data, respectively.

Table 3. Four-month post-intervention Pap smear check-up

Practice	Intervention group N %	Control group N %	P-value*
1. Pap smear uptake within 4 months			
▪ Yes	11	5	0.193
▪ No	89	95	
2. Reasons for not			
▪ No occasion	69	65	0.652
▪ No symptoms	15	24	0.530
▪ Shame	6	11	0.310
▪ Fear of pain	2	2	1.000
3. What would help			
▪ Mobile unit	27	53	< 0.001
▪ Appointment	19	10	0.108
▪ Supporting activities	17	19	0.854
4. Nothing but an occasion			
	30	19	0.100

*The χ^2 and Fisher's exact test was used for the continuous and categorical data, respectively.

Table 4. Initial and final coverage of Pap smear in both zones

Timing of Survey	Zone I N=158 N (%)	Zone II N=146 N (%)	p-value (χ^2 test)
1. Initial (Pre-intervention)	58 (36.7)	46 (31.5)	0.339
2. Final (Post-intervention)	69 (43.6)	51 (34.9)	0.119
p-value (χ^2 test)	0.070	0.374	

*The χ^2 and Fisher's exact test was used for the continuous and categorical data, respectively.

Discussion

We undertook this study to determine whether a health professional--*delivering a culturally sensitive education and invitation as an intervention at home*--could improve the cervical cancer screening-coverage rates among women between 35 and 60 years of age from the inner-city Samliem community of Khon Kaen, Northeast Thailand. We found that the rate for women in the intervention zone tended to increase from baseline to follow-up interviews with borderline significance (36.7 to 43.6%, p=0.070). Interestingly, the rate also increased among the control group over the study period (31.5% to 34.9%, p=0.374). The differences were not statistically significant in all cases except that the control group proposed more mobile unit to encourage them to get a Pap smear (53 *vs.* 27%, p<0.001). We therefore found only a marginal positive effect of the intervention on cervical cancer screening coverage rates within the intervention group.

The results are disappointing as all 200 women actually need screening according to the Thai National Cervical Cancer Prevention Strategy--*which recommends women between 35 and 60 have a cervical cancer screening test every 5 years*--and yet the time lag since their previous Pap smear was more than 5 years at the time of the survey (May, 2006). This indicates that prevention is a low priority among this population, despite their proximity to a tertiary university hospital and its community-based health station which all provide Pap smear service.

Our sample, which lives near medical facilities, should reflect the highest coverage rate for inner-city women (34.2%) compared with other areas without any intervention (5%) [5]. Moreover, this type of sample represents women who may actually be reached by health education programs when implemented in a non-research setting. Randomization of the sample resulted in nearly identical intervention and control groups. In addition to a coverage analysis using data obtained only from those subjects who completed the follow-up interviews, we conducted an analysis that included all previously excluded subjects. In this coverage analysis, we assumed that those women previously excluded still had the same screening coverage that they had reported in their baseline interviews (totally 4 months and not more than 5 years).

Our study findings, however, illustrates the need for a mobile unit even for those living nearby a hospital, since as high as 40% of respondents indicated that a proper occasion and sufficient time were the real determining factors for getting a Pap test. The two responses (1) *nothing would encourage her to get a Pap smear except the right occasion* (24.5%) and (2) *the provision of a mobile unit* (40%) perhaps explain why "no occasion" arose for 67% of the 200 women to get a Pap smear during the study period. This suggests that these Thai women were too busy to get a Pap test and that prevention is a low priority for them.

A mobile unit may be one of the best strategies for increasing screening coverage among Thai women because: (1) women think that nurses doing the procedure come from a hospital, not a health station, so feel more confident in the service; and, (2) this strategy provides an occasion for women near their home. A study conducted in rural Roi-et province, ~110 km to the east of Khon Kaen, used this strategy as a principle method for recruiting women in combination with advance appointments [17] with the result that screening coverage of women between 30 and 45 was >60% [18].

Increases in cervical cancer screening coverage rates in the control group as well as the intervention group suggest that some factors other than our intervention may have had an impact. These may have included community-wide cancer education and prevention programs sponsored by the Ministry of Public Health or the Khon Kaen Provincial Health Office and private insurance companies.

The "Hawthorne effect" may also have played a role as the baseline interview might have stimulated some participants to obtain screening tests [19]. It is perhaps not surprising that women in the control group also increased the rate at which they obtained Pap smears since the test is widely used, inexpensive, often ordered by physicians, and familiar to most Thai women [19].

Two other studies [20,21] used face-to-face education and invitations at home as an intervention; however, our result was only similar to the study by Sung et al., [20] wherein an in-home education intervention had no effect on getting Pap smears. Their study was conducted among low-income, inner-city, African-American women perhaps comparable to our study sample. By contrast, McAvoy and Raza's [21] result was that health education interventions increased the uptake of cervical cytology among Asian women who had never been tested. We suspect that the Asian women in Leicester constitute a very different socio-economic group from our sample.

We conclude that the use of culturally-sensitive, health education and home visit interventions are important. By themselves, however, these strategies are insufficient. Promoting health in developing country populations, like Thailand's, is particularly difficult because of the low priority of preventive services. Typical members of these populations are primarily concerned with their immediate needs; such that, health is a priority only in time of illness. Reaching this type of population with health promotion interventions will require additional strategies, such as: (1) sending out a mobile unit, (2) making advanced appointments, (3) using special holidays, (4) mass screening with friends, and/or (5) legislation. The key is creating opportunity.

Acknowledgements

We would like to thank Mrs. Chulaluk Na Nhongkai, a Family Practitioner Nurse at Samliem Health Station, for help doing the baseline interviews and Mr. Bryan Roderick Hamman for assistance with the English-language presentation of the manuscript.

References

[1]   Parkin DM, Pisani P, Ferlay J. Global cancer statistics. *CA: A cancer Journal for Clinicians* 1999; 49: 33-64.

[2]   British Medical Association. Cervical cancer and screening in Great Britain. London: *BMA*, 1986: 1.

[3]   Peters RK, Thomas D, Skultin G. Invasive squamous cell carcinoma of the cervix after recent negative cytology test result: a distinct subgroup. *Am J Obstet Gynecol* 1988; 158: 926.

[4]   IARC working group. Screening for squamous cervical cancer: duration of low risk after negative results of cervical cytology and its implication for screening policies. IARC working group on evaluation of cervical cancer screening programmes. *BMJ* 1986; 293: 659-64.

[5]   Srivatanakul P. Cervical cancer screening: Pap smears. In: Srivatanakul P, Koohaprema T, Deerasamee S, eds. Appropriate strategic plan in cervical cancer control and prevention of Thailand. Bangkok: *Thai National Cancer Institute*, 2000: 19-22.

[6]   Sankaranarayanan R, Budukh AM, Rajkumar R. Effective screening programmes for cervical cancer in low- and middle-income developing countries. Bulletin of the World Health Organization 2001; 79: 954-62.

[7]   Chamberlain J. Failure of the cervical cancer screening programme. *BMJ* 1984; 289: 853-4.

[8]   Chamberlain J. Reason that some screening progammes fail to control cervical cancer. In: Hakama M, Miller AB, Day NE, eds. Screening for cancer of the uterine cervix. Lyon: International Agency for Research on Cancer, 1986: 161-8. (IARC publication No.76)

[9]   MacGregor JE. Rapid onset cancer of cervix. *BMJ* 1982; 284: 441-2.

[10]   Walker EM, Hare JJ, Cooper PA. A retrospective review of cervical cytology in women developing invasive squamous cell carcinoma. *Br J Obstet Gynaecol 1983*; 90: 1087-91.

[11]   Chisholm DK, Haran D. Case of invasive cercal cancer in the North West in spite of screening. *British Journal of Family Planning 1984*; 10: 3-8.

[12]   Ellman R, Chamberlain J. Improving the effectiveness of cervical cancer screening. *J R Coll Gen Pract 1984*; 34: 537-42.

[13]   Paterson MEL, Peel KR, Joslin CAF. Cervical smear histories of 500 women with invasive cervical cancer in Yorkshire. *BMJ* 1984; 289: 896-8.

[14]   Choyce A, McAvoy BR. Cervical cancer screening and registration are they working? *J Epidemiol Community Health* 1990; 44: 52-4.

[15]   Forbes C, Jepson R, Martin-Hirsch P. Intervention targeted at women to encourage the uptake of cervical screening. *The Cochrane Library* 2005, Issue 3.

[16]   Kritpetcharat O, Suwanrungruang K, Sriamporn S, Kamsa-Ard S, Kritpetcharat P, Pengsaa P. The coverage of cervical cancer screening in Khon Kaen, northeast Thailand. *Asian Pac J Cancer Prev* 2003; 4: 103-5.

[17]   Royal Thai College of Obstetricians and Gynaecologists (RTCOG)/ JHPIEGO Corporation Cervical Cancer Prevention Group. Safety, acceptability, and feasibility of a single-visit approach to cervical-cancer prevention in rural Thailand: a demonstration project. *Lancet* 2003; 361: 814-20.

[18]   Chumworathayi B, Khunying Limpaphayom K, Srisupundit S, Lumbiganon P. VIA and cryotherapy: doing what's best. *J Med Assoc Thai* 2006; 89: 1333-9.

[19]   Gehlbach SH. Interpreting the medical literature. 3rd ed. New York: McGraw-Hill; 1993: 111-24.

[20]   Sung JFC, Blumenthal DS, Coates RJ, Williams JE, Alema-Mensah E, Liff JM. Effect of a cancer screening intervention conducted by lay health workers among inner-city women. *Am J Prev Med* 1997; 13: 51-7.

[21]   McAvoy BR, Raza R. Can health education increase uptake of cervical smear testing among Asian women? *BMJ*. 1991; 302: 833-6.

Index

2

2D, 12

3

3D, 13

A

aberrant, 45, 56, 102
abnormalities, 18, 44, 103, 108, 114
absorption, 22
academic (s), x, 62, 63, 64, 65, 69, 72, 73, 76, 78, 79, 81, 83, 86, 89, 90, 91, 92, 93, 94, 95, 96
academic difficulties, x, 62
academic problems, x, 62, 63, 81, 91, 93, 95, 96
access, 85, 95, 96
accessibility, x, 62, 94, 95, 96
accommodation, x, 62, 79, 90
accounting, 25
accuracy, xi, 100, 102, 108, 110
acetaminophen, 53, 56
acetylation, 45
acid, viii, 8, 39, 40, 44, 47, 48, 49
activation, vii, 5, 6, 9, 10, 11, 12, 13, 16, 17, 20, 44, 45, 59, 105
activation state, viii, 5
activators, 18
activity level, 10
acute, viii, 17, 39, 40, 41, 42, 44, 45, 47, 48, 49, 58
acute myeloid leukemia (AML), 41, 42, 45, 49
acute promyelocytic leukemia, viii, 39, 40, 44, 47, 48, 49
adenocarcinoma (s), vii, 5, 8, 10, 11, 13, 15, 16, 17, 101, 102, 103, 108

adenoma, 8, 58
adhesion, 20
adjustment, 64, 97
administration, 47, 80
adolescents, 97, 111
adult (s), 3, 23, 31, 32, 35, 36, 85, 101
advertisement (s), 1, 2, 94
advertising, vii, 1, 2, 3, 4
affect, 33
African-American, 122
age, ix, xi, 7, 8, 22, 23, 24, 25, 27, 28, 31, 32, 51, 53, 54, 55, 56, 67, 72, 73, 74, 77, 78, 81, 89, 93, 95, 100, 102, 113, 114, 115, 117, 120
agent (s), vii, ix, 40, 41, 44, 46, 47, 51, 56, 57, 104
age-related, 22
aging, 22, 31
aid, 103
AIDS, 4
alcohol, x, 2, 53, 55, 56, 62, 63, 69, 78, 91
algorithm, 101
alpha, 46, 47, 48, 49
alternative, 41, 101, 105, 112
American Cancer Society, 58, 109
Amsterdam, 37
analgesic (s), 53, 55
analog, ix, 39, 42, 44, 45, 46, 47, 48
analysis of variance, 10
androgen, vii
aneuploid, 105, 106
aneuploidy, xi, 100, 105, 107, 112
anger, 92
angina, 53
angiogenesis, 17, 20, 56
animal models, 56
animals, 59
anticancer, viii, ix, 17, 39, 40, 46
anti-cancer, 41, 42, 43, 44, 52
anticoagulant (s), vii, 5, 7, 10, 11, 12, 13, 14, 15

anticoagulation, viii, 5, 19
antigen, 9
anti-inflammatory drugs, ix, 51, 52, 55, 58, 59
antithrombin, vii, 5, 6
antitumor, 47, 48, 56, 59
anti-tumor, 6, 42, 43, 45
anxiety, 63, 89, 95
anxiety disorder, 63
APL, 44, 45
apoptosis, viii, 39, 42, 44, 46, 47, 56
arrest, viii, 39, 42
arsenic trioxide, ix, 40, 44, 48, 49
arthritis, 52, 53, 58
Asian, 122, 123
aspirin, ix, 52, 53, 55, 56, 58
assessment, x, 9, 18, 33, 37, 61, 63, 64, 65, 101, 105
association (s), 28, 29, 31, 34, 67
asymptomatic, xi, 100, 102
atmosphere, 94
attacks, 53
attention, 34, 90
attitudes, 93, 97
atypical, 102, 104, 112
authority, 80
automation, 109
availability, 94, 96, 111
awareness, viii, 22, 34, 90, 94, 104, 114, 119

B

Bcl-2, 42
behavior, 3, 4, 24, 33, 64
behavioral change, 2
belief systems, 86, 94
beliefs, 3, 86
benefits, 23, 93
benign, 2, 107, 111
bias, 33, 115
binding, 45, 90
biochemical, 37
biological, xi, 100, 105, 109
biology, vii
biomarker (s), xi, 100, 104, 106
biopsy, 9, 102, 106, 107
biosynthesis, 56, 59
birth, 116
blood, ix, 6, 17, 18, 19, 40, 42, 43
blot, 103
body, 47
Body Mass Index (BMI), 54
body size, 57
body weight, 47
bone, viii, 21, 22, 31, 32, 34, 35, 37, 40, 47

bone density, 31
bone loss, 32, 34, 35
bone mineral content (BMD), 22, 31, 34, 35
borderline, xi, xii, 102, 103, 114, 118, 120
brain, 40
breast, vii, ix, 20, 40, 44, 46, 48, 51, 52, 53, 54, 55, 56, 57, 59
breast cancer, vii, ix, 44, 46, 48, 51, 52, 53, 54, 55, 56, 57, 59
British, 96, 97, 98, 122, 123
bureaucracy, 62
business, 118
bypass, 66

C

calcium, viii, 21, 22, 31, 32, 33, 35, 40, 43, 46, 47
California, 2, 47
campaigns, x, 2, 3, 62, 94
Canada, 2, 63, 64
cancer (s), vii, ix, x, xi, 1, 3, 4, 5, 6, 7, 9, 14, 15, 17, 18, 19, 20, 39, 40, 41, 42, 43, 44, 45, 46, 47, 48, 49, 51, 52, 53, 55, 56, 57, 58, 59, 99, 100, 101, 102, 103, 105, 107, 108, 109, 110, 111, 112, 114, 115, 118, 119, 121, 122, 123
cancer cells, 17, 40, 41, 42, 43, 44, 46, 47, 48, 49, 56
cancer screening, 108, 109, 110, 112, 115, 121, 122, 123
capacity, 6
capital, 68
Carbon, 35
carcinogenesis, xi, 52, 56, 100, 103, 104, 105, 111
carcinoma (s), 14, 18, 101, 107, 108, 112
cardiovascular, 52, 53, 57, 58
cardiovascular disease, 52
cardiovascular system, 57
career counseling, 73, 74, 78, 83, 91, 92, 96
casting, 90
catabolism, 44, 48, 49
Caucasian, 54
CEA, 14
cell, viii, ix, 6, 19, 39, 40, 42, 43, 44, 46, 47, 56, 101, 104, 105, 108, 111, 112
cell culture, 42
cell cycle, viii, 39, 42, 46, 104, 105
cell differentiation, ix, 40, 46
cell division, 104
cell growth, 46
cell line (s), 42, 44, 46, 47
cervical cancer, x, xi, 99, 100, 101, 102, 103, 105, 107, 108, 109, 110, 111, 112, 113, 114, 115, 117, 120, 121, 122, 123
cervical carcinoma, 102

cervical dysplasia, 107, 110
cervical intraepithelial neoplasia (CIN), 101, 103, 104, 105, 109, 110, 111, 112
cervical screening, xi, 99, 100, 101, 105, 106, 107, 108, 112, 123
cervix, 100, 108, 111, 112, 114, 115, 122, 123
chemoprevention, ix, 52, 57, 58
chemopreventive, ix, 51, 53
chemotherapeutic agent, 6, 9
chemotherapeutic drugs, 46
chemotherapy (ies), vii, 5, 6, 7, 8, 9, 16, 17, 40
Chemotherapy, 6
Chicago, 47
Chinese, 48
cholecalciferol, 24, 35
Christians, 68, 90
chromosomal instability, 105, 106
chromosomes, 104
chronic, viii, 39, 42, 53, 54
chronic renal failure, viii, 39, 42
cigarette smoking, 53, 54
cisplatin, 8, 44, 48
civilian, 23
classical, 53, 104
classification, 9, 18, 111, 112
clients, 63
clinical, viii, xi, 6, 9, 17, 18, 19, 20, 22, 31, 32, 33, 34, 35, 36, 39, 40, 41, 42, 43, 44, 45, 52, 58, 63, 85, 89, 98, 99, 100, 103, 104, 106, 107, 109
clinical trial (s), viii, 6, 18, 22, 31, 39, 41, 42, 43, 45, 52, 58
clinics, 110
clone, 105
CML, 44
c-myc, 42
coagulation, vii, 5, 6, 9, 17, 18, 19, 20
Cochrane, 115, 123
cohort, 91, 101, 109
collaboration, 90, 94
collagen, 22
colon, vii, viii, 17, 39, 40, 41, 42, 47
colon cancer, vii, viii, 39, 41, 42, 47
colonoscopy, 16
colorectal, vii, 5, 12, 14, 58
colorectal adenocarcinoma, 12
colorectal cancer, vii, 5
colposcopy, 103, 106, 110, 111
communication, 3, 4, 33
community, xi, 31, 35, 66, 113, 114, 115, 117, 120, 121
community-based, 114, 121
complement, 94
complete remission, 40, 44

compliance, 33
components, 17
composition, 86
compounds, viii, ix, 33, 39, 40, 43, 45, 49, 52, 53, 57
computer (s), 88, 101
concentration, 42
condyloma, 111
confidence intervals, ix, 51, 53, 55, 67
confidentiality, x, 62, 85, 94
confusion, 4
consensus, 31, 37, 110
consent, 66
consultants, 64, 86
consumers, 2, 4
consumption, 6, 35
contamination, 115, 118
continuing, vii, 22
control, iv, ix, x, xi, 2, 4, 10, 31, 43, 51, 53, 56, 99, 104, 108, 111, 113, 114, 115, 116, 117, 118, 120, 121, 122, 123
control group, xi, 43, 56, 114, 115, 116, 117, 118, 120, 121
controlled, viii, 22, 31, 33, 35, 39, 41
controlled trials, 22, 31
conversion, ix, 40, 44
coping strategies, 96
corepressor, 45, 49
correlation, 18
Costa Rica, 109
costs, viii, 21, 22
counsel, 63, 83, 93, 95, 96
counseling, viii, x, 22, 24, 33, 36, 61, 62, 63, 64, 65, 66, 67, 69, 72, 73, 74, 75, 76, 77, 78, 79, 80, 81, 82, 83, 84, 85, 86, 87, 89, 90, 91, 92, 93, 94, 95, 96, 97, 98
course work, 91
coverage, x, xi, xii, 23, 33, 62, 100, 113, 114, 115, 117, 118, 120, 121, 123
COX-1, 42
COX-2, vii, ix, 42, 51, 52, 53, 55, 56, 57, 58, 59
COX-2 inhibitors, vii, ix, 51, 52, 53, 55, 56, 57, 58
creatine, 43
crime, 90
cross-talk, 19
cryotherapy, 123
crystalline, 40
cultural, 86, 94
culture, x, 62, 86, 91, 97
curable, 107
curriculum, 93, 94
cycles, 7, 8
cyclic AMP, 59
cyclin D1, 42

cyclin-dependent kinase inhibitor (CDKI) (s), 42, 104
cycling, 1
cyclooxygenase-2, vii, ix, 51, 52, 55, 58, 59
cysteine, 19
cytologic, 108, 110, 111, 112
cytology, x, xi, 99, 100, 101, 102, 103, 104, 105, 106, 107, 108, 109, 110, 112, 122, 123
cytometry, 100, 105, 106, 107, 112
cytopathology, 104

D

data collection, 57
database, 23, 24, 33
daughter cells, 105
death (s), 22, 52, 64, 100
debt (s), 95, 96
decision making, x, 62, 80
decisions, 80, 81
deduction, 85
deficiency, 6, 36
deficit, 11, 14, 15
definition, 9, 37
degradation, 44, 45, 49
degree, 2, 3, 54, 63, 66, 90, 101, 118
delays, 107
delivery, 24
demand, 2, 4, 73, 89, 90, 91, 92, 93
demographic (s), 23, 24, 53, 66, 67, 72, 73, 77, 78, 81, 87, 91, 95, 118
demographic characteristics, 53, 67, 72, 81, 87, 95
demographic data, 118
demographic factors, 67, 77, 78, 81, 91
denial, 91
density, 22, 31, 35, 37
dentistry, x, 62, 66, 89
dentists, viii, 22, 33, 92
depressed, 97
depression, 89, 95
depressive disorder, 63
deprivation, 3
deregulation, 56
derivatives, 7
desires, 87
detection, xi, 52, 99, 100, 101, 103, 104, 105, 106, 109, 110, 114
developed countries, x, 95, 99, 100, 115
developing countries, 65, 114, 115, 123
dexamethasone, 44
diabetes mellitus, 53
diagnostic, 101, 102, 104, 111
dichotomy, 95

diet, 22, 43
dietary fat, 59
differentiation, viii, ix, 9, 39, 40, 42, 44, 45, 46, 47, 49, 104, 111
dimer, vii, 5, 8, 9, 10, 11, 12, 13, 14, 15, 18, 20
diploid, 104, 105, 107
direct cost, 22
direct-to-consumer, vii, 1, 2, 4
direct-to-consumer advertising (DTCA) , vii, 1, 2, 3, 4
disability, viii, 21, 22
discipline, 95
discrimination, xi, 100, 103
diseases, 3, 18, 44, 52, 107, 112
disorder, 66
disseminated intravascular coagulation, 6
distress, 64, 67, 79
distribution, 23, 67, 68, 89, 102, 117
District of Columbia, 21
diversity, 86
division, 104
DNA, xi, 99, 100, 102, 103, 104, 105, 106, 107, 109, 110, 111, 112
DNA image cytometry, 107, 112
DNA ploidy, 104, 105, 112
DNA sequencing, 111
DNA testing, 102, 103, 105, 106, 109, 110, 112
doctor (s), 33, 82, 90, 92
dosage, viii, 39
dosing, 47
double-blind trial, 35
drug use, x, 62, 63, 91
drugs, ix, 1, 2, 7, 24, 39, 46, 58, 78
drying, 101
duration, x, 53, 57, 61, 66, 103, 122
duties, 93
dysplasia, 110, 114

E

eating disorders, 63, 91
E-cadherin, 42
economic, 22, 122
education, xi, xii, 54, 81, 85, 96, 97, 98, 113, 114, 116, 120, 121, 122
efficacy, 7, 22, 31
EIA, 103
elderly, 22, 23, 31, 32, 35, 36, 37, 43, 58
elderly population, 32, 36
electricity, 81, 90, 95
ELISA, 9
emotional, x, 62, 63, 75, 76, 78, 79, 83, 86, 91, 92, 94, 95, 96

employment, 72, 117
endoscopy, 9
endothelial cell (s), 6, 17, 19
England, 35, 36, 109
English, 122
Enlightenment, 84, 94
enrollment, 7
enthusiasm, 43
environment, x, 62, 66, 85, 90, 91, 95
environmental, vii
enzyme, ix, 40, 44, 51, 56
epidemiologic studies, 52, 102
epidemiological, 100
epidermal growth factor receptor, 54
epithelial cells, xi, 99, 102, 104, 111
epithelial stem cell, 105
epithelium, 104
ergocalciferol, 24, 33
esophageal adenocarcinoma, vii, 5
estimating, 24, 53, 102
estrogen, vii, ix, 52, 54, 55, 56, 59
estrogen receptors, vii, 56
ethics, 117
ethnic groups, 86
ethnicity, x, 62, 94
etiology, vii
Europe, 4, 101
European, 64, 97, 100, 108, 110
European Union, 100, 108, 110
evidence, x, 3, 17, 19, 22, 31, 34, 52, 56, 62, 64, 79,
    92, 95, 96, 99, 100, 101, 103, 105, 107, 109
examinations, 6
exclusion, 117
exercise, 94
exfoliative, 108
exocrine, vii, 5
exogenous, 53
expenditures, 23
expertise, 105
exposure, vii, ix, 1, 2, 3, 32, 42, 52, 53, 57
expression, viii, 39, 42, 44, 45, 104, 105, 111

F

facial expression, 92
factorial, 44
failure, viii, 39, 40
faith, 90
false positive, 107
family, ix, x, 26, 27, 29, 30, 32, 40, 52, 53, 54, 55,
    56, 62, 64, 77, 78, 89, 91, 92
family history, ix, 52, 53, 54, 55, 56
fat, 2, 22

fatalism, 3
fear, 85, 117, 118
feedback, 80, 81, 85, 92, 95
feeding, 3
feelings, 2, 92
females, x, 8, 27, 30, 32, 62, 72, 75, 78, 81, 87, 91,
    92
femur, 34, 37
fibrinolysis, 17
financial difficulty, 74
financial problems, x, 62, 63, 64, 92, 95, 96
financing, 94, 107
flow, 116
fluid, 109
fluorinated, 46
focusing, 32
folding, 104
Food and Drug Administration (FDA) , vii, viii, 1, 2,
    32, 39, 40, 53, 101
fortification, 32
fracture (s), viii, 21, 22, 31, 32, 34, 35, 36, 37
fragility, 22, 34
France, 1
fruits, 2
fusion, ix, 40, 44, 45, 48

G

gallbladder, vii, 5
gastric, vii, 5, 10, 11, 16
gender, 18, 23, 27, 29, 32, 63, 67, 72, 73, 76, 81, 87,
    91, 92, 95
gender differences, 63, 92
gene, ix, 40, 44, 45, 48, 56, 59, 111, 112
gene expression, 48, 59, 111
General Health Questionnaire (GHQ), 63, 66, 67, 79,
    92, 96, 97
generation, 20
genes, ix, 39, 45, 104
genetic, vii, xi, 56, 100, 104, 106
genetic endowment, vii
genetic instability, 106
genistein, 44, 48
genome, 105
genomic instability, 105
genotype (s), xi, 100, 103, 110, 111
geriatric, 32
Germany, 99, 100, 107, 108, 112
gestures, 92
God, 81, 85
grading, 9
graduate students, 97
granules, 104

Great Britain, 122

groups, xi, 18, 31, 73, 81, 86, 102, 104, 114, 115, 116, 117, 118

growth, viii, 19, 20, 39, 40, 42, 44, 46, 48, 63, 86

growth factor, 19, 20

guidance, 65, 66, 67, 69, 80, 85, 89, 90, 91, 92, 93, 95, 110

guidelines, viii, 21, 22, 32, 33, 35, 36

gynecologists, 107

H

haemostasis, 20

happiness, 80

harassment, 69, 90, 91

head, 90

headache, 53

health, vii, viii, x, xi, 1, 3, 4, 19, 21, 22, 23, 33, 34, 61, 63, 64, 77, 81, 89, 90, 94, 95, 99, 101, 102, 107, 113, 114, 115, 117, 118, 120, 121, 122, 123

health care, viii, x, 21, 23, 33, 34, 61, 63, 64, 90, 95

health care professionals, 33, 34

health education, xi, 113, 114, 117, 121, 122, 123

health effects, 3

health information, 3

health insurance, 94, 101

health problems, vii, 1, 3, 63, 77, 81, 89

healthcare, 2, 3, 34, 94, 114

height, 53

hematological, 41

hematopoietic, 42, 43, 46

hematopoietic stem cells, 42

hemodialysis, 40, 47

hemostasis, viii, 5, 6, 10, 16, 17, 18

hemostatic, 6, 7, 9, 15, 16, 17, 18, 20

high-grade intraepithelial lesions (HSIL), 102, 103, 104

high risk, 32, 103, 105, 107, 110, 112

high-risk, xi, 100, 102, 103, 104, 106, 109, 110, 111, 112

hip fractures, 22, 31, 35

histochemical, 102

histological, 53

histone, 45, 49

HIV, 4

homebound, 36

homeostasis, 40

homes, xi, 113, 115

hormone (s), 22, 40, 47, 53

hospital, 53, 94, 121

hospitalization, 41

hospitalized, 23

host, 17, 104, 111

household (s), viii, 21, 23

human, viii, xi, 4, 39, 41, 42, 44, 46, 47, 48, 49, 52, 53, 54, 56, 57, 59, 99, 101, 102, 105, 109, 110, 111, 112

human experience, 4

human papillomavirus (HPV) (s), xi, 99, 101, 102, 103, 104, 105, 106, 107, 109, 110, 111, 112

Hungary, 5

hybrid, 103

hybridization, 103, 111

hypercalcemia, ix, 39, 40, 42, 43, 46

hypercoagulable, vii, 5, 6, 17, 18, 19

hyperparathyroidism, viii, 39, 40, 42, 47

hypertension, 53

hypothesis, 3, 59

I

ibuprofen, ix, 52, 53, 55, 56, 58

identification, 18, 31, 102, 103, 104, 107

identity, 85

idiopathic, 6

imaging, 5, 7, 9, 15, 16, 18, 102

imaging systems, 102

imaging techniques, 9, 18

immobilization, 6

immunoassays, 9

immunohistochemical, 104

implementation, 100

in situ, 102

in vitro, viii, ix, 39, 40, 41, 42, 43, 45, 46, 47, 49, 104

in vivo, viii, 39, 41, 42, 44, 45, 46, 48, 49

incentive, 117

incidence, x, 3, 4, 6, 36, 63, 99, 100, 101, 108, 114, 115

income, 66, 91, 117, 123

independence, 93

indication, 3

indicators, 37, 112

individual differences, 57

indomethacin, 53

induction, viii, 39, 40, 44, 46, 47, 56, 59

industry, 2

infection (s), xi, 99, 100, 102, 103, 104, 105, 107, 109, 110

inflammation, 17

inflation, 24

Information System, 24

informed consent, x, 61, 117

infrastructure, x, 61, 65, 81

inhibition, 19, 44, 48, 58

inhibitor (s), vii, ix, 5, 6, 18, 40, 42, 44, 46, 48, 49, 52, 53, 55, 56, 57, 58, 59, 104
insecurity, 90
instability, 105, 106
insurance, 23, 24, 25, 26, 30, 31, 101, 121
integration, 104, 105, 111, 112
integrity, 44
interaction (s), vii, 6, 17, 19, 45, 49, 83
interest, 42
international, 9
International Agency for Research on Cancer, 123
Internet, 2, 85, 88, 95, 96
interpersonal relationships, 83
interpretation, 57, 101
interval, 53, 107
intervention, vii, xi, xii, 5, 57, 97, 113, 114, 115, 116, 117, 118, 120, 121, 122, 123
interview (s), xi, 53, 65, 113, 114, 115, 116, 117, 120, 121, 122
intimacy, 83
intravenous, 40, 42
invasive, xi, 53, 99, 100, 101, 102, 107, 108, 109, 112, 114, 123
invasive cancer, 101, 102
irradiation, 8
ischemic, 53
Islam, 68
isolation, 103

J

James Cancer Hospital, ix, 51, 53
January, 107
Japan, 39
jobs, 91, 94
Jun, 47
Jung, 46

K

keratinocyte, 111
kidney, 7
killing, 115
kinase, 42
King, 111
knockout, 42
kyphosis, 22, 31

L

language, 91, 92, 122
large-scale, 18

law, 97
LBC, 101, 102
lead, 3, 18, 22, 33
legislation, 122
lesion (s), 100, 102, 103, 104, 105, 107, 109, 110, 111, 112
leukaemia, 49
leukemia, viii, ix, 39, 40, 41, 42, 43, 44, 45, 47, 48, 49
leukemia cells, viii, 39, 40, 44
leukemic, viii, 39, 46, 47
leukemic cells, 46
leukocyte (s), 17, 19
lifestyle, vii, 1, 3, 63
life-threatening, 2
lifetime, 114
ligand, 44
likelihood, 29, 30, 65
limitation (s), x, 33, 82, 93, 99, 101
literacy, 3, 4
literature, viii, 21, 22, 31, 32, 34, 91, 105, 123
liver function tests, 7
location, 24, 116
London, 18, 65, 98, 122
long period, 57
Los Angeles, 39
losses, 105
Low-grade Squamous Intraepithelial Lesion (LSIL), 102, 103, 105, 107, 110
low risk, 107, 122
low-income, 122
lumen, 16
lung cancer, 20
lung disease, 53
lymphadenectomy, 8

M

macrophage (s), 42, 43, 46
mainstream, 97
males, x, 8, 27, 62, 67, 72, 74, 81, 87, 92
malignancy, vii, 6, 8, 17, 19, 43, 52, 102, 107
malignant, 6, 9, 18, 19, 105, 106, 111, 114
mammography, 53
management, viii, 21, 31, 32, 34, 36, 37, 86, 91, 95, 102
man-made, 81
mapping, 48
marital status, 72, 77, 116, 117
market, 2
marketing, vii, 1, 2, 4
marriage, x, 62, 73
mass, 108

Massachusetts, 96
measles, 104
measurement, 24, 105, 112
median, 43, 57, 103
Medicaid, 25, 27, 29, 58
medical care, 23, 97
Medical Expenditure Panel Survey (MEPS), viii, 21, 23, 24, 25, 26, 27, 28, 30, 31, 32, 33, 36, 37
medical school, 97, 98
medical student, 63, 64, 74, 87, 96, 97, 98
Medicare, 27, 29, 37
medication (s), viii, ix, 2, 9, 18, 21, 23, 24, 31, 33, 34, 51, 53, 55
medicine, x, 1, 26, 27, 28, 29, 30, 32, 33, 35, 62, 66, 80, 86, 89, 110
men, 23, 25, 32, 34, 35, 36, 37, 63, 85, 92
menopausal, 32, 53, 55, 56
menopause, 22, 23, 35, 55
menstrual, 53
mental health, 62, 63, 64, 89, 90, 92, 93, 94, 95, 98
mental health professionals, 63, 89
messages, 2, 3
meta-analysis, 109
metabolism, 40, 46, 57
metabolite, ix, 40, 44
meta-message, vii, 1, 2, 3
metastasis, 6, 7, 18
metastatic, 6, 18
mice, 42, 44, 48
microenvironment, 22
microscopy, 102
military, 112
milk, 35
mineralization, 22
minority, 93
misunderstanding, 64
mitochondria, 44
mitochondrial, ix, 40, 44
mitogenesis, 56
mitosis, 105
modalities, 105, 107
models, 3, 67
modernization, 37
modulation, 18
molecular weight, 40
molecules, vii, 20
money, 81, 95
monocytes, 6
mononuclear cells, 6
mood, 97
moral standards, 85
morbidity, 4, 6, 63, 64, 67, 79, 92, 97
morphological, xi, 100, 103, 106

mortality, x, 4, 6, 35, 41, 52, 99, 100, 108, 115
mortality rate, 52, 101
mothers, 82
motivation, 65, 91
mucus, 101
multiple myeloma, viii, 39, 41
Muslims, 90
mutagenesis, 56
myelodysplastic syndromes, 47
myeloid, ix, 40, 41, 42, 44, 46, 48
myeloma, viii, 39, 41, 42, 44, 47
myocardial infarction, 52, 53, 58

N

nation, viii, 21, 89
national, viii, 21, 22, 23, 24, 25, 27, 31, 33, 117
National Academy of Sciences, 4
National Institutes of Health, 22
natural, 10, 11, 12, 14, 15, 18, 22
needs, 105
neoplasia (s), xi, 100, 101, 102, 103, 105, 107, 109, 110, 111, 112
neoplasms, 52
neoplastic, xi, 6, 100, 104, 111
networking, 94
neutropenia, 9
New England, 35, 109
New York, 21, 57, 58, 123
New Zealand, 3
newspapers, 90
Nigeria, x, 61, 65, 68, 86, 89, 90, 91, 94, 95, 97, 98
non-institutionalized, viii, 21, 23
non-small cell lung cancer, 20
non-steroidal anti-inflammatory drugs (NSAIDs), ix, 51, 52, 53, 55, 56, 58
non-urban, 25
normal, ix, 4, 11, 14, 15, 16, 18, 40, 43, 46, 102, 104, 111
normalization, 11, 12, 14, 16, 17
North America, 36
Northeast, xi, 25, 26, 27, 28, 29, 30, 69, 113, 115, 120
nuclear, 49, 104
nuclei, 105
nucleus, 105
nulliparity, 54
nurse (s), viii, 22, 33, 64, 74, 91, 94, 97, 98, 121
nursing, x, 62, 64, 66, 67, 82, 87, 89, 91, 94, 97, 98

O

obligation, 89
occupational therapy, 64, 96
odds ratio, ix, 25, 51, 53, 55, 56, 74, 79, 87
office-based, 23, 24
Ohio, ix, 51, 53
older adults, 32, 35
oncogene (s), 44, 48, 49, 105, 111, 112
Oncology, 39, 58, 59
oncoproteins, 104
online, 99
optimization, 22
oral, 6, 7, 19, 35, 43, 47
organ, vii, 5, 7
organization, 62
orientation, 94, 96
orthodox, 90
osteoarthritis, 53, 58
osteocalcin, 22
osteopenia, 34
osteoporosis, viii, 21, 22, 23, 24, 28, 30, 31, 32, 33, 34, 35, 36, 37
osteoporotic fractures, 34, 37
out-of-pocket, 94
outpatient, 94, 109, 110
ovarian cancer, 53, 54
over-the-counter (OTC), 33, 53, 55

P

paclitaxel, 44, 48
pain, 22, 53, 117, 119, 120
pancreas, 18
pancreatic, vii, 5, 13, 14, 15
pancreatic cancer, 14, 15
Pap, x, xi, xii, 99, 101, 102, 103, 106, 109, 110, 113, 114, 115, 117, 118, 119, 120, 121, 122
Pap smear, xi, xii, 101, 102, 103, 110, 113, 114, 115, 117, 118, 119, 120, 121, 122
Papillomavirus, 111
parameter, 18
parathyroid hormone, 22, 47
Paris, 19
pathogenesis, 44
pathology, 53
pathophysiology, 22
pathways, 6
patient care, 24
patients, viii, ix, 2, 4, 6, 7, 9, 10, 11, 12, 13, 14, 15, 17, 18, 19, 20, 21, 23, 24, 25, 27, 28, 29, 30, 31,

32, 34, 37, 39, 40, 42, 43, 44, 45, 47, 51, 58, 103, 104, 111, 112
PCR, 103, 104, 106, 110, 111
peak concentration, 42
peer support, 94
peers, 89
pelvic, 119
Pennsylvania, 1
peptide, vii, 5, 6, 9
perception (s), 3, 69, 79, 97, 98
performance, 7, 9, 98, 105
periodontitis, 37
peripheral blood, 43
permit, 2, 107
personal, 33, 53, 64, 65, 81, 83, 93
personal history, 53
personal life, 64, 83
personality, 93
perspective, 33, 36, 100, 109
pharmaceutical ads, vii, 1
pharmaceutical companies, 2, 3
pharmaceuticals, vii, 1, 2, 4
pharmacist (s), viii, 22, 24, 33, 36, 37
pharmacotherapy, 36
Philadelphia, 1, 18, 36
phosphate, 22
phosphorus, 40, 47
physical activity, 2, 22
physical health, x, 62, 79
physicians, viii, 22, 23, 24, 28, 29, 30, 32, 33, 36, 121
physiological, 64
physiotherapists, 91
physiotherapy, x, 62, 66, 67, 73, 74, 78, 87, 89, 91
pilot study, 98, 115
placebo, 31, 34, 43
planning, 89, 91
plasma, 20, 42
plasminogen, 18
platelet (s), 6, 17, 19, 20, 43
platelet count, 43
play, 23, 57, 83
ploidy, 104, 105, 112
plurality, 80
poison, 59
polymerase chain reaction, 110
polymorphism, 110
polyp, 52
polyploid, 105
polyploidy, 105
poor, viii, 21, 43, 44, 95, 101

population, viii, 2, 3, 21, 23, 25, 26, 31, 32, 34, 36,
    41, 58, 63, 64, 67, 86, 97, 100, 101, 102, 103,
    105, 107, 108, 109, 110, 114, 115, 117, 121, 122
postmenopausal, ix, 22, 23, 34, 35, 36, 52, 54, 55, 56
postmenopausal women, ix, 23, 34, 35, 36, 52, 55,
    56
postmortem, 6
postoperative, 16
Postpartum, 119
powder, 40
power, viii, 39, 115
prayer, 90, 97
precancerous lesions, 100
preclinical, 56, 63
predictors, viii, 21, 30, 32, 37
pre-existing, 53
preference, 64
pregnancy, 6, 53
premenopausal, ix, 52, 55, 56
premenopausal women, ix, 52, 55
premium, 94
preoperative, 16, 17
preparation, 89, 91
prescription drug (s) 3, 4, 37
prevention, vii, viii, 1, 2, 3, 4, 21, 22, 24, 31, 32, 33,
    34, 35, 46, 58, 99, 105, 121, 122, 123
preventive, vii, 64, 122
primary care, 4, 23, 33, 66, 97
privacy, 85
private, 25, 31, 85, 121
probability, 24, 33
probe, 103, 110
procoagulant, 6, 18, 19
profession (s), x, 37, 61, 63, 64, 90
prognosis, viii, 5, 6, 43, 104
prognostic marker, 7, 18
prognostic value, 18, 105
program, 37, 66, 93, 94, 100, 106, 115, 117
progressive, 10, 12, 13, 14, 15, 112
proliferation, viii, 39, 46, 47
promote, vii, 1
promoter, 44, 59
promyelocytic, 44, 49
prophylaxis, viii, 5, 35
prostaglandin, ix, 51, 56, 58
prostate, vii, viii, 20, 39, 40, 41, 42, 43, 46, 47, 48,
    49
prostate cancer, vii, 20, 42, 43, 47, 48, 49
prostate carcinoma, 20
protection, 114
protein (s), vii, ix, 5, 6, 9, 19, 22, 40, 44, 45, 48, 49,
    104
prothrombin, vii, 5, 6, 9

protocol (s), xi, 7, 8, 100, 102, 103, 107
proximal, 59
PSA, 43, 47
psychiatric disorders, 66
psychiatrist (s), 85, 94, 98
psychiatry, 63, 91
psychoactive, 91, 97
psychological distress, x, 62, 63, 65, 66, 67, 79, 90,
    91, 96
psychological problems, x, 62
psychological stress, 63, 92
psychologist, 83, 85
public, xi, 3, 23, 31, 99, 101, 102, 107
public health, xi, 3, 99, 101, 102, 107
P-value, 118, 119, 120

Q

quality control, 57
quality of life, 4
questionnaire (s), ix, x, 51, 53, 62, 66, 67, 89, 115,
    117

R

race, ix, 1, 23, 25, 28, 30, 31, 51, 53, 54
radiation, vii, 5, 8, 41, 49
radiological, vii, 5, 18
radiologists, 9
radiotherapy, 8
random, 53, 115, 117
randomized controlled clinical trials, 41
range, 2, 9, 42, 43, 69, 101, 104
rat (s) 46, 48, 59
reading, x, 99, 117
reagents, 9
recall, 52, 53, 57
receptors, 56
recognition, xi, 65, 99
recreational, 81
recruiting, 121
recurrence, 52, 102
reduction, ix, 15, 22, 31, 45, 52, 55, 56, 57, 63, 101,
    114
reflection, 90
Registry (ies), 57, 108
regression, xi, 25, 28, 32, 53, 67, 73, 74, 76, 77, 78,
    79, 87, 100, 105, 110
regression analysis, 32, 53, 78
regression equation, 73
regular, ix, 22, 52, 53, 94, 95, 100, 114
regulation (s), vii, 1, 2, 57

regulators, 104

reimbursement, 103

relationship (s), 6, 18, 20, 63, 64, 65, 67, 73, 79, 81, 83, 86, 87, 89, 91, 92, 93, 95, 97

relatives, 54

relevance, 94, 115

reliability, 27

religion (s), x, 62, 68, 72, 90

religious, x, 62, 86, 90

religious beliefs, 86

remission, 1, 49

renal failure, 40, 42

repression, 45

repressor, 45

research, vii, 3, 4, 31, 52, 57, 63, 64, 92, 105, 121

researchers, xi, 1, 22, 67, 95, 113

resection, 8

residual disease, 102

resources, viii, 21, 93, 114

restriction fragment length polymorphis, 110

retinoic acid, viii, 39, 40, 44, 47, 48, 49

retinoic acid receptor, 48, 49

returns, 2

rheumatoid arthritis, 53

risk, vii, viii, ix, xi, 3, 4, 6, 21, 22, 31, 32, 37, 51, 52, 53, 55, 56, 57, 58, 63, 92, 99, 100, 102, 103, 104, 105, 106, 107, 109, 110, 111, 112

risk factors, vii, ix, 51, 53, 56

risk profile, 103

RNA, 104

rofecoxib, ix, 52, 53, 55, 56, 57, 58

rural, 89, 115, 121, 123

RXR, 44

S

sales, 2

sample, viii, 9, 21, 24, 25, 36, 53, 98, 101, 118, 121, 122

sample survey, 98

sampling, 24, 25, 33, 101, 110

school, 64, 65, 80, 83, 85, 96, 97, 98, 118

school authority, 80, 85

scores, 66, 79

screening programs, x, 99, 100, 101, 107

search, 104

secretion, 47

secrets, 83

security, 90

segregation, 105

selecting, 103

selective estrogen receptor modulator, vii

selectivity, 40

self, 26, 27, 29, 103, 110

self help, 95

self-report, 95

SEM, 54

sensitivity, x, 62, 66, 99, 101, 102, 103, 104, 105, 107

separation, 62

sequencing, 106, 111

serum, 41, 43, 46

services, x, 3, 23, 34, 37, 61, 64, 65, 86, 90, 92, 94, 95, 96, 97, 98, 122

severity, vii, 47

sexual harassment, x, 62, 78, 90

shame, 117

sharing, 80

short-term, 58

side effects, 2

signalling, 48

signs, 9, 34, 104, 106, 109, 111

single test, 107

sites, 9, 34

skeleton, 22

skills, 63, 94, 95

skin, 40

smoking, 53, 55, 56

social, 33, 63, 64

society, 90

software, 25

solid tumors, 18, 19, 46

solutions, 2, 82

somatic cell, 104

specialists, 29, 30, 32

specialization, 86, 91

specificity, x, 66, 99, 101, 102, 104, 105

spectrum, 111

S-phase, 105

spiritual, x, 62, 77, 79, 85, 86, 90, 94, 95, 97

squamous cell carcinoma, 112, 122, 123

St. Louis, 35

stability, 54

stages, 52, 64, 86, 104

stakeholders, 37

standard error, 25

Statistical Analysis System (SAS), 25, 58

Statistical Package for the Social Sciences (SPSS), 67

statistics, 105, 122

statutory, 100

stem cells, 46, 105

steroid hormone, 40

stigma, 64

stomach, 16

strategic, 122

strategies, 90, 101, 112, 117, 121, 122
stratification, 55, 103
stress, x, 61, 63, 64, 66, 79, 80, 81, 82, 91, 92, 93,
   96, 97, 98
stress level, 63
stressors, 64, 96
stroke, 53
student group, 73, 95
students, x, 61, 62, 63, 64, 65, 66, 67, 68, 69, 72, 73,
   74, 75, 77, 78, 79, 80, 81, 82, 83, 84, 85, 86, 87,
   89, 90, 91, 92, 93, 94, 95, 96, 97, 98
subgroups, 56
subjectivity, 102
substance use, 91
substances, 6, 18
Sunday, 97
supervision, 94
supplemental, 22
supplements, 37
supply, 81, 90, 95
suppression, 40, 49
suppressor, ix, 39, 104
surgery, vii, 5, 6, 8, 9, 16, 17, 21, 31, 53, 107
surgical intervention, 9
surgical resection, 8
surveillance, 102, 107
survival, 41, 47
symptoms, 6, 64, 102, 117, 119, 120
syndrome, ix, 39, 43, 47
synergistic, 44
synthesis, 6, 58
synthetic, viii, 39, 40
systematic review, 108, 115
systems, vii, xi, 5, 17, 46, 64, 99, 101, 102, 103

T

tamoxifen, vii
target behavior, 3
target population, 66, 67
targets, vii
teachers, x, 62, 77, 80, 82, 90, 93
teaching, 82, 93
technology, 103
telephone, 2
television, vii, 1, 2
telomerase, 104
tension, 92
terminally ill, 115
territory, 68
testicular cancer, 1
Thai, 115, 117, 121, 122, 123
Thailand, xi, 113, 114, 115, 120, 122, 123

theory, 4
therapeutic, ix, 9, 19, 22, 23, 40, 46, 47, 57, 80
therapeutic agents, 19, 47
therapy, viii, ix, 19, 22, 25, 27, 28, 29, 30, 31, 34, 35,
   36, 37, 39, 40, 43, 44, 48, 52, 54, 107
thinking, 3
threshold, 66
thrombin, 6, 9, 19, 20
thromboembolic, 7, 19, 58
thromboembolism, viii, 5, 6, 19
thrombosis, 6, 18, 19, 20
thrombotic, 58
time, vii, 1, 2, 3, 10, 11, 12, 13, 14, 53, 56, 57, 58,
   62, 66, 67, 83, 85, 86, 89, 91, 92, 93, 110, 117,
   121, 122
tissue, 18, 19, 104, 105
tobacco smoking, 2
Tokyo, 39
toxic, ix, 39, 40, 43
toxicity, ix, 40, 43, 46
tracking, 23, 32
training, 63, 64, 82, 85, 92, 93, 94, 95, 96, 98
trans, viii, 39, 40, 44, 46, 48
transcript, 112
transcription, 44, 49
transcriptional, ix, 22, 40
transformation, xi, 47, 100, 104, 105, 106, 111
transfusions, 43
transition, 63
translocation, 44, 49
transport, x, 62
treatment programs, 22
trend, 11, 12, 16, 27, 32, 73, 76, 90, 95
triage, 102, 105
trial, ix, xi, 35, 39, 40, 42, 43, 45, 58, 110, 113, 115
trust, 83
tubular, 17
tumor (s), vii, ix, 5, 6, 7, 8, 9, 15, 16, 17, 18, 19, 39,
   42, 43, 45, 46, 49, 52, 55, 59, 101, 104
tumor cells, 6, 17, 18
tumor growth, 6
tumor progression, viii, 5, 18
two-way, 10

U

undergraduate (s), x, 61, 62, 89, 91, 92, 97, 98
uninsured, 26
United Arab Emirates, 5
United Kingdom (UK), 31, 63, 65, 94, 95, 96, 98
United States, 53, 64, 85
univariate, 67, 72, 74, 77, 87
universities, 64, 65, 95

university education, 62
university students, 62, 63, 91, 95
urban, 25, 26, 29, 30
users, 23, 25, 27, 28, 32, 94

V

vaginal, 110
validity, 66
values, 8, 9, 10, 18, 27, 28, 29, 30, 33, 43, 79, 101
variable (s), 14, 24, 29, 32, 53, 55, 56, 67
variation, 36
vascular, 17, 18
vector, 45
vegetables, 2
vein, 20
venue, 85
victimization, 83
Vioxx, ix, 52, 53, 57, 58
viral, xi, 99, 110
virological, 105
virus, 105, 106
visual, 105, 112
vitamin D, viii, ix, 21, 22, 23, 24, 25, 26, 27, 28, 29, 30, 31, 32, 33, 34, 35, 36, 37, 39, 40, 41, 42, 43, 44, 45, 46, 47, 48, 49
vitamin D deficiency, 32
vitamin D receptor (VDR), ix, 39, 42, 44

W

Wales, 36
Washington, 4, 21, 35

water, 90, 95
web, 2
wellness, 97
wild type, 42
women, ix, xi, 22, 23, 25, 30, 31, 32, 34, 35, 36, 52, 53, 55, 56, 63, 85, 93, 100, 101, 102, 103, 104, 105, 107, 109, 110, 111, 112, 113, 114, 115, 116, 117, 118, 120, 121, 122, 123
words, 27
workers, 123
working hours, 85
workload, 63, 64
World Health Organization (WHO), 9, 114, 115, 123
worry, 63, 107
writing, 66

X

xenografts, 42

Y

young women, 109, 110

Z

zinc, 45